Firmly In His Hands

Firmly In His Hands

smugs and hooches, Dink

Alan Coleman

Writer's Showcase
San Jose   New York   Lincoln   Shanghai

Firmly In His Hands
smugs and hooches, Dink

Writer's Showcase
an imprint of iUniverse, Inc.

For information address:
iUniverse, Inc.
5220 S. 16th St., Suite 200
Lincoln, NE 68512
www.iuniverse.com

ISBN: 0-595-22512-8

Printed in the United States of America

This book is dedicated to the hundreds of generous souls who left their footprints on our beach.

Epigraph

This sickness will not end in death.
—Jesus Christ, John 11:4

Contents

Acknowledgements

Virginia Palmour: Thank you for asking that question. And for responding so positively to my initial attempts to find its answer.

Catherine Parnell: Thank you for saving Dink's words and generously sharing them with me.

Jean Burton: Thank you for suggesting I turn my "writings" into a book.

Len Strozier: Thank you for keeping me accountable as the manuscript developed.

Susan Fahncke: Thank you for 2theheart.com and its readership family who showed me that Dink's legacy is far from over.

Ann Spillers: Thank you for finding the errors in the manuscript that I would have sworn were not there.

Carla Ferry: Thank you for convincing me to quit waiting on other people to make it happen.

Sara, Joe and Sam Coleman: Thank you for not giving up on me when I should have been looking for a job instead of sitting at the computer for so long.

Introduction

I Couldn't Answer Virginia's Question

It all started as an attempt to answer a question a young friend of mine asked. She had lost a close and dear friend in an automobile accident and she said to me, "I miss Rob so much. How do you deal with losing your wife?" On any given day, when anyone asked me that question, I would usually reply with the old standard, polite but trite, "One day at a time." But I could hear a genuine pain in Virginia's words and I could tell she needed a genuine answer rather than some socially acceptable brush-off. That's when I realized I didn't actually know how to answer her question. I told her I would try, but it would take some time because I had not yet thought completely through the answer in my own mind, let alone verbalized it to anyone.

I started by giving her a brief synopsis of our experience with the disease. It was the first time I consciously looked at what we had gone through from start to finish. I went back to some emails I wrote early in April 2000 because I remembered how they reflected my frame of mind at that point in time. I added some background and explanation to each message, being very careful to think through the words thoroughly because I knew I had to state them in a way a nineteen-year-old could understand. I began emailing these thoughts to Virginia, telling her that maybe the answer to her question would present itself—to both of us— over time.

To: Alan
From: Virginia
Mon Aug 28 2000

Hey Alan,
Well I guess the party was a success. I had a great time. It was a good thing I left when I did because it took me about 3 hours to finish my homework. Oh well…. When are you going to be down this way or should I say up this way? I get out of classes on Tuesdays and Thursdays at 11:50. We could do lunch on those days. So how are you doing? I have had a hard weekend. I miss Rob so much!!!! I just can't stand it. It really isn't fair for anyone. Can I ask a personal question? Well I am going to anyway, but you don't have to answer. How do you deal with your wife being gone? How did you prepare for that and what helps you get through it (besides having people like me and Phyllis in your life)? Well it is getting late and I am probably boring you. I hope to see you soon. Have a great day! God is watching over us all.
Virginia Claire

To: Virginia
From: Alan
Wed Aug 30 2000

I'm sorry the weekend was tough on you. I never knew Rob, but I've gained a tremendous amount of respect for him over the last few weeks. I consider myself less of a person for not knowing him. You wrote: "How do you deal with your wife being gone?" It may take a while before I can answer your question. Not from an emotional standpoint, and certainly not from being hesitant to talk with you, because I'm not at all, but from the standpoint that I'm not sure of the truthful answer. I don't want to respond to you with the polite but canned, socially correct, "One day at a time," like I would tell most other people who might ask. I'm trusting that you want the real answer and that's what I intend to give you. I just don't have a total handle on it yet. I'll probably have to send you a series of "stuff," all of which together, might yield the best answer. You answered a large part of it yourself: God, and people like you and Phyllis. Let me start by giving you a little background on what happened. My wife's name was Debra, but her family nickname was Dink, so that's what I've always called her. She was diagnosed in January of 1998, with amyotrophic lateral sclerosis, or ALS, also known as Lou Gehrig's Disease. Within 6 months, she could no longer speak, and she couldn't eat or drink by mouth. At the end of 1998, she began losing strength in her arms and shoulders. In the Spring of 1999, she began having walking problems and by that fall she was in a wheelchair. By mid-January of this year, she was 100% dependent on a caregiver. She passed away—I call it her Day of Victory over the disease—on March 28, less than two weeks before Phyllis and Rob's accident. I think the first part of the answer to your question is actually contained in an email I sent to a friend a few days after she died. I'll track it down and forward a copy to you. Hope you haven't opened a bigger can of worms than you imagined. If I get long winded, bear with me...I am a teacher, ya know.

later gator,
Alan

Over the next few weeks, I sent Virginia a series of email messages, attempting to find the answer to her question. It wasn't long before I realized this process was helping me, probably more than it was helping Virginia. Then I remembered all the emails Dink had sent to me. For no specific reason, they had never been deleted, so I began applying the same process to them. It was a gut wrenching, emotional, cleansing, therapeutic, heart breaking, uplifting, touching, astonishing, enlightening, encouraging, restorative process and it's the single-most beneficial thing I have experienced since Dink has been gone.

This book is the result of that process. It contains a compilation of email and fax messages Dink wrote between September 1998 and December 1999. I've left her words essentially unedited, except for spelling corrections, as I didn't want to paraphrase her thoughts and risk losing the humor that makes her, and these messages, so special. As explanation and background, I've added my own thoughts to most of the "topics of the day," but many of them need no input at all from me.

SEPTEMBER 1998

These Things Take Time

To: Big Al
From: Dink
Date: Wed 30 Sep 1998 06:28
Subject: Good morning, stud muffin

Hi,
My eyes weren't open yet when you left so I thought I would say Good
Morning. The sleeping medicine you gave me was too wonderfully
strong. We'll have to work on the dosage a bit. These things take time
and patience and lots of trials. But I know we can achieve success,
together.

Go Team!
Lugs and Hisses,   _____ and _____   *(Look on page 203)*
DC

*Dink always tried to be awake to tell me "Goodbye" in the mornings, but so
many times that deep sleep just before dawn was the most effective for her
and thus the most difficult to wake from. So the morning interactions we
traditionally had while getting ready to go to work were replaced by emails
she would send to me later in the day.*

Because of the disease, sleeping restfully and regularly had already become a challenge so we embarked on a number of experiments and trials to overcome that challenge. We tried a variety of medications that are supposed to cause drowsiness. We experimented with a ton of different sleeping positions, including the use of an assortment of pillows to prop various body parts. We even lowered the foot of the bed a few inches, which resulted in both of us waking up crunched against the footboard—humorous, but not very restful. We tried the "coma couch," so named because it was known to induce coma-like naps on Sunday afternoons, even claiming each of the kids on various occasions. When we would discover an effective solution, and finally get some consistent rest, it would only be temporary because the disease would take another progressive step and introduce new sleeping challenges.

It's remarkably appropriate that this was the first of our "AM Ems"— Morning Emails—which I happen to have saved. It reflects so much of what came to be the theme of our fight against ALS: time, patience, lots of trials, and most importantly Teamwork.

OCTOBER 1998

Our Foundation of Communication

Date: Mon 05 Oct 1998 06:41
Subject: TOUGH DECISIONS

I know last night was hard for you, but you had lost your faith in it and you have never been able to promote something you thought to be unethical—except Team Flamingo. I'm glad we sat together to come up with that decision. Now we can put our attentions elsewhere.
Other hard decisions of late:

      Getting out of bed this morning
      Getting off the couch to take Sam to 500 church activities
      Putting on that tie this morning
      Leaving me this morning—with my wompy hair and monster breath

I know I won't see you tonight until you bring the princess home so know that I love you forever. Unwaveringly. (Actually it's the sex) Have a terrific day and make a difference in someone's life.

You go, Grand Nim/poop! I'll see you tonight. Be thinking about which book you want to read tonight. Much lubs.

With ket wisses,   *With _____ _____*
Dink

We had been involved with a multi-level-marketing business and I decided to bail on it. MLM's are a lot like Communism: in their pure and uncorrupted form, everybody wins. The problem with both arises when you introduce people into the equation. I had recently discovered that the leaders in our particular business were making as much money on the business building supplies they sold to their organization as they were making on the consumer products being distributed to retail customers. More importantly, that profit was being misrepresented to the organization, so we told our partners we were resigning. That was the hard part because our partners were, and still are, our good friends (who happened not to be in the big money either). One of the good results of that affiliation was our relatively new commitment to doing more reading and less "televisioning." We even got Sam to join us occasionally. How about that…Mom, Dad and Teenager sitting in the den reading together. It's pretty cool.

Sara, our oldest at 25, was the first born granddaughter on the Hobby side of the family. She was the little girl her grandmother Myrtis never had, and she received all of Myrt's pent up doting, so Dink occasionally referred to Sara as "the princess." Having graduated from college earlier that summer, Sara was living at home again, looking for a job in Atlanta. Our other two kids are boys. Joe is 23, and Sam is 18.

Team Flamingo and Grand Nim/poop are references to a group of guys I used to do a lot of bicycle riding with. As one of the Founding Flamingoes, my team title was Grand Imperial Nincompoop…and that's really all that needs to be said about that.

Date: Tue 06 Oct 1998 06:36
Subject: UMMMMM…..

My head wasn't even cranked into slow gear this morning when you left. It's like…you got up and were instantly dressed, then gone!

It's about 6:30 and Sam's alarm just came on. It'll be another 30 minutes before he starts moving. And Sara will start moving about that same time. Then we all rush out the door at the same time, 7:40.

I liked the format last night—9pm, reading, together. I think I might want to add a dimension. Occasionally add a topic for discussion or talk about some aspect of our work or house or marriage or kids that may need attention. Although all are perfect and I could never see any aspect of trouble in any.

Well, this is a short note, I have to get in gear. I checked our email and had a poem from Bec Christian and a lousy joke from Aubrey.

With smugs and hootches, (an oldie but goodie)
_With _____ and _____
Dink

One of the things that attracted me to Dink back in 1980 was the ease with which we could talk. She and the kids lived across the hall from my apartment and I met her for the first time when I knocked on her door to ask if I could borrow her newspaper to look for another place to live. One of my roommates had left for Colorado, the other was transferring to another college and I was way too broke to afford the apartment alone. We talked at her door for several minutes then she asked if I wanted to sit down and we spent the next two hours sitting in her den talking about everything in the world. The conversation didn't always come that easily through the years, but I'm convinced the foundation of communication we started building that day is what allowed us to overcome the obstacles we faced later on. The significance in this message is that she had long before lost the ability *to speak. She communicated through the use of an electronic device that could speak the words she typed. It was laborious and slow and occasionally hard to understand, but she never hesitated to "say" what was on her mind. At the end of the disease, it was the last thing she could still do by herself.*

Date: Wed 07 Oct 1998 07:03
Subject: Yawn….

Good Morning Sunshine Babee…
I found a time when Sam nor Sara are on the telephone! WOW!

Not much to say this morning. Just finished my shower and it is 6:55 so I'm running late, again. But I got one load of clothes on and I unloaded and loaded the dishwasher so I'm on a home-roll.

I forgot to tell you to be careful driving so if you are reading this at school I guess you're covered by yesterday's declaration.

We need to insert a little dancing time into our nightly plans, occasionally. The Beatles are singing "Twist 'n' Shout." That's where that thought came from.

Although you didn't have your tie on yet, you were working on a very hot look today. Make those women keep their hands off My babee.

I will see you tonight at the church, with bells on. Figure how else I can help you stay afloat, I'm ready, willing, and able. Enough for now, Sam just got up. I love you mightily.

Big, long sloppy kiss,
Dink

Date: Thu 08 Oct 1998 06:33
Subject: HIYABABEE
Good Thursday morning, sweet thang,

I'm sitting waiting for the iron to warm up. I just woke Sam up so I'm pretty sure my life is in danger.

Whatever came over me last night, I'll call "Having to watch Dawson's Creek, Pizza Guys and Girl, because the Braves were in rain delay." No let's be honest—Sara and Sam are bigger than me!

Sara left it at "I'll get back to you" as to where she wanted to eat. So I am thinking maybe Don Pablo's in Conyers, if they are open. What do you think?

Well, Sam's up, and not speaking. I think I'll make a run for my cozy room—oh, but, I have to iron first—drat! Gotta go!

Rack bubs & meet fassage,   _____ _____ & _____ _____
Dink

Dink loved the Atlanta Braves, even before they became the "Team of the Nineties," and would watch them nightly. Sam used to watch them with us until the strike of '94, after which he called them "money suckers" and started a personal boycott. Sara never did care much for watching them on the tube, so we had regular "discussions" about what to watch since we only have one television. I guess Dink had relinquished the TV to the kids that night because of a rain delay in the Braves game and ended up watching some of her least favorite shows. We should have been reading.

For the last several years, one of our family traditions has been to let the kids choose where we would eat on their birthdays. Sara's ambivalence was *concerning Dink because this message was sent on the morning of Sara's birthday and we still needed to coordinate with Joe, who would have to drive over from Athens to hook up with us.*

Date: Fri 09 Oct 1998 06:39

I LOVE YOU.

Dink

Geez…what can I say?

Date: Fri 09 Oct 1998 05:58
Subject: YO!

I was just getting the "Ken" email to forward and decided to email you, too.

You are in the shower right now and I could be wicked and turn on the washing machine (it's loaded and ready), but it's Friday and I wouldn't want to destroy that fragile mood Friday gives us.

Sam has the game tonight, I'm sure Sara is busy, too. We could take Ken to see "Ronin," or go out to eat or tour Covington, or……now it's your turn to figure out entertainment.

Well, you are out of the shower so I will go accost you (and start my washing machine).

Much lubs and kisses,
(I'm straight today),
Dink

Ken Christian is one of Dink's cousins and, in a way, is responsible for these archives. He lives "up north" and had long been only a name to me, but he came into our lives in a large way about a year before this message. It seems as youngsters, Ken and Dink did not get along fabulously because Ken had discovered she was a fairly easy target for an assortment of good-hearted bullying and he availed himself of every opportunity to make her a victim. As an adult though, he was struck with a huge case of guilty conscience, and resurfaced in our lives to make an honest attempt to make amends with Dink. Ken earns his living as a "computer guy" which is a title I give to anyone who can make one of these things be profitable. On one of his visits he was bemoaning the fact that we didn't have email. On the next visit, he showed up with his old computer which had been replaced by his new computer and told us it (the old one) would work fine for emailing. He gave us the computer and hooked us up with an email service and promptly got Dink hooked on e-talking to everybody. I'm sure it seemed to Ken that he was just doing one of his "computer things," but I will always be grateful to him for introducing this communication medium to us. It made a huge difference in Dink's life.

Date: Tue 13 Oct 1998 06:43
Subject: Mornin' Glory

Late night last night, but much more fun than it could have been. I still have the sleepies this morning.

We'll have surveyors at the hospital the next three days. Everyone is in a twit. Competition for the secretaries' time and talents with graphs. Clean, clean, clean! Then clean some more! This is just a "mock" survey. Joint Commission comes next November. We pay these folks to come in and get us ready.

I haven't been in Medical Records since last Thursday. I hope I have Kathy ready enough that I can spend some extra time in Medical Records—and with the lab project. Someone was complaining yesterday that it was unfair that Kathy had a "Debra"- that everyone needed a "Debra."

Enough of that, remember Sam's committee meeting tonight.

Gotta go get showered. Thanks for shaking me this morning. Have a stupendous day, and don't let them take you hostage. Go Get'em!

Hugs and Kisses,
Dink

The "Joint Commission" is the accreditation agency for health care services in Georgia. Passing their assessment is a stressful event that takes a ton of preparation by everybody in the hospital. Newton General Hospital, where Dink worked as an RN, hires an independent consultant to stage a "mock" Joint Commission visitation to help them evaluate their preparedness. This trial run is almost as stressful as the real thing.

Having lost the ability to communicate traditionally in the clinical setting with patients, families, and doctors, Dink was moved into a position that could be categorized as quality assurance. Every hospital would love to have someone with her clinical expertise in that capacity, but few can afford to pull such a person away from direct patient care. She absolutely excelled, making contributions in a wide variety of departments around the hospital. I can remember her bemoaning the fact she had been requested in more places than she could fit into her schedule. In fact, it created a bit of a challenge for the Human Resources department to keep up with which hours of her salary were to be charged to which department. Probably her proudest moment professionally came in January of 1999

when she was named NGH Employee of the Year for 1998. It's so wonderfully ironic that something which would typically be considered a diminished capacity could lead to such a valuable and exemplary contribution to
the success of the hospital.*

Date: Thu 15 Oct 1998 06:28

Good morning!

This is a very short one because it's prayer breakfast day. I had to
shorten my "zone."

I am so looking forward to having you all to myself, even if it's only for
32 hours. It'll be fun.

Like last time, I was convinced the ALS was affecting other areas of my
body. Any time I can't open something with my left hand, or when I
stumble over something, that gray cloud sneaks in, but I know not to
worry, this will go where it wants to go and we'll just "handle it."

Well, gotta run, before the "prince" awakens. Now we have the prince
and the princess at home. Wow! Enuff—

Snuggles and squeezes,
Smackee face!
Dink

*Prayer Breakfast is a prayer meeting for the youth of our church that is
generally held at a local restaurant before school on Thursdays. For Dink
and Sam, that meant leaving the house 30 minutes early, but I don't think
they ever got out of bed 30 minutes early, so they were always rushing more
than usual on Thursday mornings.*

I guess she felt like Sam needed equal time in the royalty references she had been giving to Sara.

"That grey cloud" was just beginning to cast its long, dark shadow. Up to this point in time, you wouldn't know she was sick if you didn't need to communicate with her. She was still doing everything that anybody else was doing—except whispering during church—but then we started seeing the first signs of large-muscle-group involvement in the disease. There were two signs I remember vividly. She was sitting on the floor, leaning back against the couch, and tried to push down on the couch with her left arm to initiate a standing movement. The look in her eyes told me she couldn't do it. A short time later we were out at the local water reservoir on one of our "walk-n-talks." The reservoir is a beautiful 800-acre lake with a public park and is protected by strict usage controls. Being free of the intrusive sounds of motor boats and jet skis, it's a wonderful place to spend time and had been our favorite walking location for years. It was on one of these walks that her left toe snagged the ground a lot more than usual. Not enough to cause her to trip, but enough to be noticed. We loved being at the reservoir so much that we never spoke of this, though we both knew what it meant. As far as I can remember, regarding the disease, that was the only denial in which we ever allowed ourselves to indulge.

Date: Thu 15 Oct 1998 13:57

Are you about ready to leave? I have packed all but your jeans/pants and shirts. If you're gonna be very long, call me and tell me how much to take out of the bank, I have to run to town to refill one of my medicines at Kmart.

Call!
Dink

Without looking back in my calender, I can tell you we had an appointment in Charlotte, NC, at the Carolinas Medical Center (CMC) on Friday, October 16, 1998. I can tell that by the date and tone of this message. When it was time to get down to business, Dink didn't waste a lot of useless words. She was obviously getting antsy about the trip.

We had been traveling to Charlotte since very early in the disease. The first local neurologist we saw was what you might call a "general neurologist" and he immediately referred us to a neuro-muscular specialist in Atlanta. We visited the Atlanta doctor for the second time in November of '97 and left that day with an appointment to return on January 14, 1998. We were still in the "can't rule out ALS" stage of diagnosis, so Thanksgiving, Christmas, and New Years were all quite a strain as we tried to deal with the uncertainty we faced. At the January appointment, Dr. Jeffrey Rosenfeld told us he was 99% sure Dink had ALS, but not to hang any hope on the 1% possibility she did not. By this time we knew why he said that.

Diagnosing ALS is a very difficult matter because there is no disease-specific diagnostic test for it. Instead, you are tested for a host of other diseases and if all of those tests turn out negative, then it is assumed with 99% certainty you have ALS. Part of the excruciating reality at this early stage in the disease is having to wait a longer period of time for more symptoms to develop before you can be 100% sure of the diagnosis. Luckily, the treatment does not have to wait. Dr. Rosenfeld started Dink on a very aggressive regimen of powerful drugs whose purpose is to slow the progression of the disease. He then advised us that when we returned for our next appointment, we would be seeing a different doctor because he was moving to Charlotte.

WHAT!?!? Do you have any more good news for us? What we were thinking was, "You can't leave us!!" but what we asked very politely was "Why

Charlotte?" Although it was only our third visit with Dr. Rosenfeld, we were impressed and touched by his calm, caring manner and had fully adopted him as "our" doctor. We couldn't believe he would already abandon us, especially without consulting us first! He explained that CMC was setting up a multi-disciplinary ALS clinic and had offered him the directorship. What he had was an opportunity to go from being a small fish in a large pond to being a large fish in a HUGE pond. He told us the clinic would be staffed by more than a dozen specialists from different areas of expertise so patients would get comprehensive assessment and treatment during each visit there. We looked at each other and then back at him and asked, "Can we go too?" He had to be diplomatic and bureaucratic with his answer because he couldn't give the appearance of "taking" his patients to his new hospital, but essentially he said, "Yep." In April of 1998 we made the first of our 25 trips to Charlotte and began falling absolutely in love with the place.

Date: Mon 19 Oct 1998 07:41

Mornin' still no wallet gotta GO!

LUBS N' MORE LUBS
Dink

What dead-head stoops to stealing a wallet from the purse of someone who works in the hospital where one of his own relatives is being cared for?

Date: Thu 22 Oct 1998 06:58

GOOOOOOD MORNING, ALAN COLEMAN!

How's life right about now. I'm moving very slowly. A bit cold blooded this AM.

Now don't take this too seriously. I had the most incredible 6 of the last 7 days. I thoroughly enjoyed spending that time with you. You are truly wonderful. I'm a lucky girl.

Enough! Enough! OOey GOOey alert!!!!

No one is up here, yet, except me. I've washed my hair but haven't combed it yet so I look pretty scarey. It was very welcome: seeing the snuggle bear last night. This morning while you work on stuff and drink your coffee, know you are cradled in the love of so many people—I personally know of hundreds—and let yourself feel that in each sip of coffee you take this morning—because you better not be drinking that stuff after lunch.

Oh! I'll stop. My head is getting cool so I'll jump back into the swing of the morning. (You stay cool yourself though, baby)

Buggle Snunnies,   _____ _____
Dink

Date: Fri 23 Oct 1998 07:35

It's FRIIIIIIIII-day!!!!!!!!!!!!!!!!!!!!!!!!!!!!!!!! Boy! These two days in a row are tough! Let's be careful out there.

The list for me on the bathroom detail is 20 long and growing. I hope to have it cleared out for you by in the morning.

Sorry this is late. I am actually on time and only did a little zone—too cold outside the bathroom to run around in my tee shirt.

Well, everyone else is up—battle of the radios and fight for the ironing board and hot water. Not too bad, no fussin' this morning, I don't think they're awake.

OK, I'm gone, but then you've known that for a while now. You are rubbing off in spots. Have a stuporous day and I'll see you this afternoon.

(It's Friday, I'm all out of ideas)
Lubs,
Dink

We had recently taken on a project we had been talking about for a long while. Actually, it was one of those projects we had talked about for years. You know the kind of project I'm talking about, especially if you're married. It's the kind that's so small and easy you've become embarrassed to talk about it because you know it should have been completed a long, long time ago. Anyway, we were finally going to repaint our bathroom and put a decorative border up at the ceiling. Now for some world class rationalization: I'm glad we procrastinated on the bathroom project because I think it was more fun as a diversion from the disease than it would have been as a plain ol' project. I'm pretty sure she'd roll her eyes at that line of thinking and say, "Oh, Al...puh-LEAZE!"

Date: Mon 26 Oct 1998 06:36

Well, it's Monday! Time renewed! Another chance to make a difference in those precious little minds. Go forth and conquer.

I just can't stand it. No spooning last night and precious little snuggling. Was it.......your nose? Or did I have b o? We'll have to work on that. I have to have adequate snuggle factor in my blood before I can face all those pining for a hug.

The dishwasher is going, the washing machine will do the same soon, the eggs are cooked, but I haven't showered or done my 45 things a female does after the shower and medication taking. I'll sprint for the clock again today. But it is so nice in the afternoon not to have to expend my subtotal energy on those things. This afternoon I think folding clothes might be in order.

I'll go now. I feel better after talking to you. Have an exceptional day to start off an amazing week. I love you more each day in new and wonderful ways and areas.

Dink

Dink had gone through quite a transformation in the last several years and I think the disease served to accelerate and accentuate those changes. In the early years of our marriage, she had not been what you would call a "people person." She shied away from groups of people, preferring to be alone or with just the kids and me. She sometimes even had a hard time being comfortable when we would get together with our respective immediate families.

This always struck me as really strange because she was such an outstanding nurse. She could get crotchety old men and women to totally relax and cooperate when other nurses and doctors seemed only to agitate them. She was known for doing small things like mini-massages that would go beyond medical protocol and add tremendously to the patients' comfort. She seemed to have a natural knack for recognizing the anxiety a new nurse felt and she would take this person under her wing and make sure they had a successful entry into the profession. It seemed like the professional uniform validated her in some way that social life did not.

In the past few years though, she began to change and it all started with her hugs. She had always been aware of the power of a hug and at some point she began giving hugs to her older patients when they left the hospital. Then she decided there was no reason to wait until they left the hospital so she began giving them hugs as part of her nursing care. Hugging the patients lead to hugging their families, many of whom already thought she was wonderful because of the high level of personal comfort she tried to achieve for their loved one. Hugging the older patients also lead to hugging the senior volunteers at the hospital which lead to hugging other staff members. I can remember going to the hospital to eat lunch with her, long before she was sick, and it would take ten minutes to walk to the cafeteria because she had to stop and hug everyone we saw along the way. As all of this was developing, we began seeing former patients and their families around town and of course a hug-fest would ensue. Then it got to the point on Sunday mornings that we would have to get to the church sanctuary early so she could go around the entire room and give nearly everyone a hug. About this time, people started talking about "Dink's Hugs." "Have you had yours today?" they would ask each other. We would always be the last ones to leave church because people would line up to get another hug.

She began calling all of this her "Hug Ministry" and it's absolutely amazing how effective it was. Earlier in the fall of the year that she wrote this message, we were shopping at a local grocery store. The lady at the cash register was relatively new at that store and was having a tough time getting products to scan properly, so it was taking her a long time to get each person checked-out and on their way. You could see the frustration and even embarrassment building on her face as her line kept growing. Then we stepped up and she had a hard time understanding Dink's communication device, so I know she felt bad about that too. When she totaled our groceries, the debit card machine malfunctioned and it was painfully obvious the poor lady had reached her last straw. Very calmly, Dink stepped around the check-out counter, which unnerved the lady a bit more, then gave her a huge hug. The lady's entire affect was transformed. You could literally see her change as she released a deep sigh and exhaled all of those pent up frustrations. Unable to say a word, Dink had truly ministered to this lady and absolutely made her day. I don't know how many other strangers Dink may have hugged before she was no longer able, but I'm still astounded that those hugs, as well as all of the others she gave, were being given by a person who at one time wouldn't even make eye contact with most of the people she met.

Date: Tue 27 Oct 1998 06:54

Oh me. Oh my. I'm moving so slowly. I took a bubble bath and it slowed me down. But I am through with the water here at 6:45 so the lazy bones can't fuss at me today.

Prior to the bubble bath I was treated to the most succulent spoonage. It was delicious in a snuggle kind of way.

Well, Salt Shakers is canceled for tonight. What do you want to do instead? We have to do something. Somewhere. Don't we?

I'll ponder on that today. Probably it is a good night to catch up on reading and folding clothes and, maybe, break out those flannel bed sheets.

Nibbles and nuzzles,
Dink

"If the truth be known..." That phrase usually precedes something a person might not otherwise readily admit. Of course, here in the South we shorten it, as in, "Truth be known, Dink and I have a natural lazy streak in us." Which is actually quite true. Everything else being equal, there's

nothing we would prefer to do more than curling up in bed and spooning the day away. Especially when the weather was cool enough to put flannel sheets on the bed. It's the last day of October 2000 as I write this and the weather is calling for flannel sheets. There are a million things I miss about Dink, but spooning is very near the top of the list.

Salt Shakers is an informal fellowship program at our church. It's pretty neat. The names of all the couples that sign up are randomly assigned to groups of four. One couple hosts dinner for the other three couples and provides the meat dish. Each of the other three couples brings either veggies, bread and drinks, or dessert. The groups are reassigned for each of the next three months, so at the end of the rotation, each couple has had dinner with twelve other couples. Hopefully, most of the twelve couples would be people you didn't already know, so you would have the chance to get to know people you don't normally get to spend time with at church.

Date: Wed 28 Oct 1998 06:40

Boy do I feel gross. I haven't taken my shower yet and my hair is wompy and I have that "been used" feel to my body. But a shower will clear up all of that.

I am getting really very excited about this research study. Kinda giddy. Thank you so much for handling everything. You are a rock.....and a fine specimen at that. I don't know just how much to tell the kids until we see if I qualify. Maybe just go through the first visit for tests. And then cover the implant after that? I just don't quite feel what's right yet.

If you want me to I will send a letter to Dr. Hadden and let her know what is going on and ask her forgiveness for taking you away so often. I'll even send flowers if you think she would like that.

Anyway, I'm babbling. Gotta go jump in the shower and use up all the hot water so S & S will have something to talk about.

Swug and hack,   _____ and _____
Dink

During our July '98 clinic visit in Charlotte, Dr. Rosey told us about a new clinical drug trial that would be starting in November. ("Dr. Rosey" was Dink's pet name for Dr. Rosenfeld. The nick-name came about partly out of affection, but mostly because it was a good email short cut.) The study was not for a new drug, but for a new method of delivering a drug that was already in use. As in most trials, a placebo would also be involved, so only two-out-of-three participants would actually receive the drug. In fact, it would be a "double-blind" study, which meant even the good doctor would not know who was receiving the actual medication. He warned us that a serious but routine surgery would be involved and we would have to start traveling to Charlotte monthly rather than quarterly and for all our trouble, it would be possible that even if she got the actual medication, it might have no effect on the disease. He told us to think about it a few days and if we determined we had an interest, to call and set up an appointment to come back for tests to see if she qualified to participate. We made the appointment before we left that very day.

Dr. Hadden was my assistant principal who had the thankless job of securing substitutes for absent teachers. By the end of that school year, I had been absent nineteen or twenty times...over ten percent of the year. Dink knew the challenge we were presenting to Dr. Hadden and though she didn't send flowers, she did send a very nice card. Dr. Hadden stopped me later and said she had never received a "thanks and apology" card from a teacher, much less a spouse, and was very touched at Dink's thoughtfulness for others. That thoughtfulness had become Dink's forte'.

Date: Fri 30 Oct 1998 07:17

FRIDAYFRIDAYFRIDAYFRIDAYFRIDAYFRIDAYFRIDAYFRIDAY
FRIDAY
TGIFTGIFTGIFTGIFTGIFTGIFTGIFTGIFTGIFTGIFTGIFTGIF
TGIFTGIF

UNDERSTAND?

LUV YUH, MAN!
Dink

PS: SORRY SO LATE

NOVEMBER 1998

The Clinical Drug Trial

Date: Mon 02 Nov 1998 07:03
Subject: Mornin'

So what did you put in my sleepin' medicine? Down for the count 2 or 3 times. Man!

Well our Bartlett pear tree right outside the study window has shades of gold and orange ablazin'. Looks like we may have our own personal show.

I am sending an email to the Northwestern ALS study that Gary's mom told us about up in Charlotte (she emailed me last night). I typed it up last night and will send it when I send yours to you. I think Mom and Daddy will let me take a little blood for a good cause. At least we'll see.

I should have told Mom I was glad to bring the cakes home, but couldn't I have some vegetables and ham? But, they don't need to be eating cake. Of course neither do we. But we can dispose of it "out of view" from Mom.

Well, someone caused me to oversleep this morning and I am behind. I do have breakfast cooked and my uniform ironed and my medicine mixed and stewing. Now comes the shower. I hate to get in the shower when my feet are cold and they're cold this morning. But good cheer, mate! Here I go!

Buzzles and kaby nisses,   _____ and _____ _____
Dink

One of the encouraging things in the world of ALS is the huge amount of research being conducted around the globe. The Northwestern study she is referring to is concerned with those instances where ALS occurs within the same family. Actually, only five percent of all ALS cases are familial, but the hope is that a causal connection can be made between family members with the disease, which could lead researchers to the general cause.

Dink's Mom is one of those Southern women whose home you never leave without taking some kind of food and, since her Dad was diabetic, Dink didn't argue about bringing the cakes home. I guess now I'll have to face my mother-in-law to explain "disposing out of view." I love my mother-in-law…she's the best. ('Reckon that'll help?)

Date: Tue 03 Nov 1998 14:38

Hey!
It's 2:30 and I had to run home and put roast in the crock pot. I forgot again this morning. My routine is such a disaster in the mornings, I need to write one up and follow it. And include other stuff to do before I walk out the door.

I know ya'll all went out for lunch. I hope it was delicious and lot's of fun. Don't get the snoozies this afternoon.

Well, better run back. I don't want to—it is simply gorgeous outside. I need my hammock back in the tree so I can sway and sleep to the rocking of the breeze. Oh, well…..Gotta go—

Hooches and smugs (an oldie but a goodie), _____ and _____
Dink

Teacher work day—wahoo! The most significant implication of a teacher work day is that we get to take an hour to go out and eat lunch…just like real professionals.

Date: Wed 04 Nov 1998 07:02

Good Morning Sweetie,
I have my lunch and breakfast packed, and all my drool managers. These are the things I have forgotten 1 day or another. It's the last 20 minutes that get me. Once I see it is 7:20, I have to go in Zoom Zone so I lose focus on planning the rest of the day.

Make sure, that you are sure, that you will be able to work Friday. If I get through at 5 and we have afternoon traffic and supper to deal with, it may turn into a 6 or 7 hour drive. Anyway, I'm gonna leave my work appearance hanging in the balance.

I am excited and very nervous about this testing tomorrow. The PFT is mostly on my mind. I KNOW my lungs are in good shape, but there is no way I have figured out to seal this big 'ole mouth of mine. But then you probably have 10 or 12 ideas about that. Maybe it's time I heard them, they might help.

Well off to the shower, before the onslaught of kids invade my peace and quiet. I love you ENORMOUSLY!!

Rear akin wug bishing,   _____ _____ _____ _____
Dink

On those rare occasions that you can drive from our house to Charlotte without stopping for gas, food, or potty breaks, you can get to the medical center in a tad over four hours, assuming also it's the right time of day, you have perfect weather, and you manage to avoid the state troopers. For some strange reason, if any one of those conditions is not met, it takes forever to get there—or to get back home. Since I had decided not to take Friday off, she's making sure I am aware we will most likely be getting back from Thursday's trip well after midnight. We were going to Charlotte to see if she qualified for the clinical trial.

One of the hallmarks of ALS is that it progresses in different ways and at different rates in different patients. Two patients can be diagnosed at the same time with similar onset symptoms, which would lead you to think they would have similar progressions, but one might lose function of his legs, then his arms, and reach the end of the disease quickly while still being able to talk clearly. The other might progress slowly, losing arm function first then surviving for many years without the ability to speak.

The one symptom that could be considered truly "common" in the disease is the loss of pulmonary function caused by failure of the diaphragm. PFT is a method of testing lung strength that involves blowing into an airflow measuring device, and it was the primary qualifying test for the clinical trial. Dink was concerned because her lips lost their muscularity early in the disease and had been hanging limp for quite some time. She knew she could not form a tight seal with her lips around the PFT device and the escaping air would falsely reflect a diminished lung capacity. When we got to Charlotte and expressed concern about this to Dr. Rosenfeld, he told us he shared the same concern and had approached the company sponsoring the trial about using an alternate testing method. Since participant testing had already begun in other trial locations, the company could not allow any variations because doing so could compromise the results of the study. So we got creative.

When it was time to do the PFT, we practiced several different "lip sealing" techniques before taking the actual test. We found a towel that was just the right size, when flattened out and then rolled up, that it could be circled around her mouth to form a seal. So, in went the PFT mouthpiece, then the towel was positioned and the nosepiece was put on. As she blew into the device, I used both of my hands to apply pressure on the towel all the way around her mouth. Another person was holding the nosepiece in place to make sure my fat fingers did not dislodge it, and another was operating the PFT machine. It took four of us, including Dink, to do what normally takes two, and we had to do it a number of times to get it right, but we made it work. She qualified with readings just above the minimum threshold, but she qualified nonetheless.

Date: Fri 6 Nov 1998 09:08
Subject: HI

Alan, this is Dink,
Do you have Dr. Rosenfeld's and Ruth's email address with you. If not where is it?

Dr. Stillerman wants it to get a faxed copy of the study Prospectus (what they are doing)

I'm using Valorie Patrick's computer at work so email her or call Ann at 770xyz4311.

I love you,
Dink

Dr. James Stillerman has been our local family doctor for longer than I can remember and he is nothing less than a saint. When Dink first realized there was something wrong, she stopped Jim at the hospital one day, just to let him know she would be calling his office to set up an appointment to see him the next week. He asked what was wrong and when she told him, he immediately took her into the first empty room he could find and did a preliminary exam. Rather than seeing Dink the next week, he referred her directly to a local neurologist.

Throughout the duration of the disease Jim was constantly double checking to make sure the staff at Charlotte was doing this or trying that. He remained Dink's primary care physician, treating the usual stuff that arose besides the ALS, including a thyroid problem she had had for years. When we would visit him in his office, he would always greet her, of course, with a hug. After the official poking and prodding and "How does this feel?" and "Does that hurt?" he would remove his stethoscope then slide his stool forward so he could look her right in the eyes. Then, holding both of her hands in his, he would ask, "What else can I do for you?" He asked that question every visit and every time he asked, I could hear in his voice and see on his face the anguish of knowing he couldn't do enough.

As is the custom here in the South, on the night before Dink's memorial service, we had "visitation" at the funeral home. As Jim came through the receiving line, he was visibly shaken. When I took his hand, it was trembling and his eyes revealed that he was searching for, but couldn't find the right words to say, so I said to him, "She always trusted you completely." I felt it was the greatest compliment I could give him, both professionally and personally.

Date: Mon 09 Nov 1998 06:52

Hi!
It's Monday morning. ARGHHHHHHHHHH.

My goal is to get everything else done and be in the shower by 6:45. I'm a few minutes late. I have b'fast and lunch packed and a load of clothes washing, but I hadn't written you my morning love letter and I couldn't live with myself if I missed it again!

The weekend was nice. And the yard looks great. Although you got sore, being out in the glorious weather did your soul some good. Even though your sinuses didn't follow that lead.

Sara came in last night, immediately got on the computer. How do I know that? Her keys are right by the keyboard. Our communication media addict.

Enough dribble. You have to get ready for the enem…I mean students. Have a fabulous day.

Love,
Snuggles

Once upon a LONG time ago, I was a fairly decent athlete. I was never a star at anything, but I could participate in almost any sport without shaming myself…except golf. Regardless of the sport being played or how well I did, though, I was never sore the next day. I would never have guessed that raking leaves could be so brutal to a person's body. How embarrassing.

Date: Thu 12 Nov 1998 06:58

Hi Sweetie,
I got to thinking about something you said last night. I think tonight I
will move something out of the study and move a comfortable chair in
so I can sit and read while you get frustrated. Especially since
"Thunder" is on tonight and I don't want to sit and listen to the good
natured but teeth-grindingly annoying banter.

Well it's 6:52 and I'm ready but Sam is just getting out of the shower.
HA!

I can't believe there are 2 more full days of work before a day or two off.
Maybe if you talk to Sara about Thanksgiving, your reasoning skills will
work better on her than mine did. I thought I was just trying to keep her
informed so she wouldn't say, "Nobody ever told me that!"

Enough. I want you to have the most amazing day. Somewhere, someone or something will cause you to be amazed.

I love you, eternally….and even tomorrow,
Dink

*We've never been "formal living room and dining room" kind of people, so
what was intended to be the dining room when our house was built has
gone through a variety of incarnations including TV room, sewing room,
office and finally, study. We never actually liked the name "study" because
it sounds rather stuffy, but it's a lot better than "the room where the computer is." I know just enough about computers to get myself in trouble with
them and whatever I was attempting to do with ours at this point in time
was evidently not going too well. I guess she decided to sit with me and my
frustration at the computer rather than with Sam and his frustration at*

his favorite wrestler's defeat. (Who would ever have thought in the 1960's that "Live Atlanta Wrasslin" would take the entire nation by storm in the 1990's?)

Date: Fri 13 Nov 1998 06:36

MMMMMMMMMMMMMMMMMMMMMMMMMMMM MM.............MMHI,

I just can't get it in gear. BUT IT'S FRIDAY!FRIDAYFRIDAYFRI-DAYFRIDAYFRIDAY FRIDAYFRIDAYFRIDAY YIPPEE YIPPEE!

Don't forget we have 5th quarter tonight. Did you call Nancy Mock last night? You were sequestered in the study for a WHILE. Any progress? I don't know when you came to bed, but I was tossing and turning until you got there.

IT'S FRIDAYFRIDAYFRIDAYFRIDAYFRIDAYFRIDAYFRIDAY.

Do you think getting some of the hardware for the computer will help with the new toy? I thought that's what you were going to do first. Please sir, I just don't understand, sir.

I had exactly 6 Granny Smith apples for the dessert tomorrow night. But the Sara machine ate one last night so I guess I'll have to buy one more, unless they get hit again before tomorrow afternoon.

I'm trying another way to cook my hard boiled egg. I have been having trouble with them breaking during boiling, so I read my good old "has everything in it recipe book," *The Joy of Cooking*. I'm following the recipe and it takes about 20 minutes at different heating levels. So I'm writin' you and checkin' the eggs. But I also need to iron my uniform so

I'll have to leave you. Parting is such sweet sorrow…but I'll be late for work. I luv ya, man!

Yetching and strawning,   _____ and _____
Dink

Date: Sun 15 Nov 1998 20:42

internet—southwest airline—buy 1 get 1 free

She had been after me for quite some time to go out to Albuquerque to visit my sister. I finally made it, with Sam in tow, in October of 2000.

Date: Mon 16 Nov 1998 14:27

It's about 2:20 and I'm home. I kept getting a tickle in my throat, coughing, drooling, nose running, then I would start wheezing and freak everyone out.

After 3 times in 30 minutes, I gave up. I decided to come home and medicate heavily and zone out. I hope it works.

Drive safely on the way home. It is still wet out there. I love you, HeMan.

lubs and sneezes,
Dink

Looking back at Dink's entire experience with the disease, by far the worst symptom she had to deal with was not a symptom of the disease at all. It was sinus drainage. That sounds preposterous, doesn't it? Since she could not control her swallow reflex, when she would have sinus drainage, it would usually get stuck in the back of her throat. That would cause a laryngeal spasm which usually lead her into hyperventilation. Because the disease had achieved full bulbar involvement, not only were her lips, tongue, and swallowing affected, but the muscles that controlled her vocal cords were weakened too, so any unusual passage of air through her throat would cause a sound of some sort. (I can't count the times she embarrassed herself by releasing a deep sigh in church, which would be accompanied by a loud, involuntary vocal response, to which she would react by covering her mouth with her hands…and blushing quite noticeably.) "Wheezing" is much too mild of a term to describe the sound she would make when she hyperventilated. It was an unnerving, strangling, penetrating sound with alarming volume. It scared me to death the first time I heard it and, in fact, scared her to death the first time it happened. It was always startling to anyone who had never heard it before.

We eventually learned through experience that she could control the spasms by taking long, slow, deep breaths. Usually she could do it without help, but sometimes she would need encouragement or a little coaching if the spasm was particularly bad. We developed one of those "communicative gazes" so when a spasm started, I would stop what I was doing and look at her and she would let me know with her eyes whether she had things under control or needed some help. If she needed help, I would hug her loosely from behind so she could feel my chest against her back. Then, with my cheek near her ear so she could hear my exhales, I would take long, deep, exaggerated breaths. Almost naturally, she would match her breathing to mine and in a few moments the spasm would subside. Most of the time, after she began breathing normally again and before I would release her from my hug, I would give her a big kiss, right on the ear, then tease her about the goose bumps that would instantly appear on her arms. (I never could resist the urge to flirt with her a little.)

One of the things we both found humorous was the concerned looks I would get from strangers when she had a spasm in public, and would control it herself while I sat nearby, appearing to be unconcerned. Their unspoken words were always, "Aren't you going to DO something!?!" On one occasion, a rather indignant lady did not leave the words unspoken.

Date: Tue 17 Nov 1998 06:33

Mornin' Sweetie,

I slept significantly better last night. I took another dose of Nyquil around 3 and could get into a position so I didn't honk, until this morning after the alarm went off the first time.

I don't think I'll go to work today either. I am still pretty wheezy when I cough and it gets embarrassing for me to be such an attention-getter. But I know they all are showing me their care and concern.

Also, it will give some time to do a few things around here that I may not feel like doing after Friday. I'm trying to be as prepared as I can. I feel lists coming on!

I hope you got a superior grade on your observation yesterday. You should get one any day they come in your class to see what you have done with your babysitting classes. You da'man, man, honey, dumplin'.

We now have a battle of the morning music alarms. Sara's about scared me to death Sunday morning. It was SO loud and I couldn't find any of the switches in the dark. I'll get Sara or Sam to call Catherine to tell her I won't be there. Today I'll try to stay busy and not lay around and maybe my body will start fighting back better. Remember to eat lunch and a late afternoon snack and I'll try to have something delicious and piping hot for you. But if you are going to be really late, go ahead and eat supper, too. I don't want you to eat supper about 9.

Well, let me close. I'm starting to cough and that messes up my typing.

Snips and nuggles,   _____ and _____
Dink

The big day was approaching rapidly. We were going to Charlotte on Friday, November 20, for the clinical trial surgery. The drug involved in the study was a synthetic form of a naturally occurring substance called brain derived neurotrophic factor, BDNF, and its job is to strengthen nerves at the spinal column, protecting them from degeneration. It is hoped that supplementing the naturally occurring BDNF will help to slow the progression of ALS. It's been studied before and showed no effect, but that was when applied by injection into the muscles. The difference in this study is that BDNF would be applied directly on the "roots" of the nerves within the spinal column. There would be around 270 participants in the study at twenty–four locations world-wide, and Dink was excited because she was going to be "patient number two" in the whole world.

Date: Mon 23 Nov 1998 06:49

Mornin',
Thought I might not have as bad a headache today and in fact until I got out of the shower I didn't have any pain. But it is back now. I "drank" the coffee, thank you, and crushed up some ibuprofen this time to see some possible difference. I WILL beat this!

Thank you so much for the shower assist-ance. My body virtually tingles! I can't tell you how tempting you were all snugged up and all that and all that this morning! You were totally distracting to my sleep activity!

I have another expansion of an idea you've already had for the ALS notebook. I'd like to develop a way to "graph" my strengths, times and reflexes, and the PFTs. This will give me a way to see where I'm headed and get a rein on it before it catches us unprepared. When I woke up about 3:15 to go to the bathroom, I stayed awake about an hour just thinking. You had virtual electrons flying around you in the bed laden with ideas and "STUFF"....and you slept through the whole thing.

Well, I'll go. I know I have gotten you tired already. I hope your Monday is a great one. I hope after four–and–a–half days away you haven't lost your touch. I am such a lucky person to have such a wonderful person to share my "eventful" life. And I don't believe anyone else could have played the part you have for the last year with the care and teamwork approach you have brought to this opportunity we have been handed. Like Bo says, "You've been given an opportunity....DO something with it." And you and I, have.

I love you immeasurably,
Dink

The surgery went extremely well. It lasted nearly three hours and went off without a hitch. Dr. Rosenfeld's administrative assistant, Sandy Wilkinson, sat with me in the waiting room the whole time. We talked about everything under the sun...except politics and sports. She is one of the sweetest and most caring people I have ever known. Since that day, I feel like I have a new sister.

The details of the operation are simply amazing. Dink was given a medication pump that continuously delivered the BDNF through a small tube directly into her spinal column. The amazing thing is that the entire delivery system was IMPLANTED in her abdomen. The pump was placed in her right front side and the tube was "fished" around from there, just below the skin, to get to her spinal column. After the surgery, the only evidence that any of it was there was the bulge in her tummy that was made by the pump. She later joked about becoming the bionic woman.

The operation also involved a spinal tap which causes unpleasant consequences. Because spinal fluid is actually withdrawn during a spinal tap, the reduced volume of fluid remaining in the spinal column will almost always lead to a delayed, but enduring headache. The headache can be reduced somewhat by remaining flat on the bed for several hours after the procedure, but since most people don't feel the discomfort immediately, they make the common mistake of getting up and moving around too soon. As a nurse, Dink had seen this happen to patients a number of times, so she was very compliant when the doctors told her to stay in bed after the surgery. We found out later that many of the other study patients were not, and a few of them had to spend an extra night or two in the hospital because of the severity of their headaches. Over the course of a few days, the spinal fluid will replenish itself and the headache gradually goes away. She was still waiting for that to happen.

The first step of her "bionic" conversion occurred in April of 1998. At that point in time, she could still talk somewhat and was still eating and drinking by mouth, but the doctors told her she would eventually need a feeding tube, commonly called a "PEG." A PEG is simply a tube that enters the abdomen through a small incision and provides direct access to the stomach. They encouraged us to consider getting one before she actually needed it, so by the time she did need it, she would already be comfortable using it. When they suggested a time frame within the next few months, we said, "How about next week?"

The PEG procedure was much less involved than the pump implant. It took place at NGH, in the out-patient center, so we were home by noon of the day it was done. Within the week, we were using the PEG for medications and hydration. That's why she said she "drank" the coffee, because she actually ingested it through the PEG. She also mentioned in an earlier message that her medications were "stewing"—we had to make sure they were completely dissolved before pouring them through the PEG so it would not become clogged. Eventually, all of her intake was via the PEG. I remember the emotional blow she took the first time we were at a restaurant and she did not order anything because she could no longer eat. We spoke later of being thankful the PEG had become second nature by that point so we were not having to learn how to use it at the same time we were facing that emotional challenge.

That pro-active attitude became one of the hallmarks of our fight against the disease. We were determined we would do as much as we could, as early as we could, to be prepared for the changes we knew were going to happen. I'm convinced that doing so reduced any feelings we may have had that the disease was "happening to us." On the contrary, we were determined we were going to happen to the disease. She refers here to the "opportunity" we had been handed. We became so accustomed to "doing something with it" that before long, she started calling it "Our Great Adventure."

Date: Mon 23 Nov 1998 10:42

Hey, Sweetie,
It's just past 10:30. I am medicated well. The aching is right behind my eyes and waxes and wanes.

Rita emailed back. Erin and Steve have a new car so they will be at her house for Thanksgiving and she laid out your mother's plans.

Mark Weaver emailed, too and I replied with a long letter—yes, I included the kitchen sink.

The phone has rung twice. Once 4 times and once 8 times. I did my own call-in this morning to Catherine's voice mail—after 3 tries. But I was persistent and PREVAILED! I am intoxicated with my own power!

Powerfully Yours,
Dink

Mark Weaver was the first patient in the world to get started in the BDNF study. We met him in Charlotte when we were there for the implant surgery. He was there to get his pump filled for the first time, having had the surgery a month before Dink. Mark had been a golf pro at a country club in Sumter, South Carolina, and his wife Marion is an elementary school teacher. Over the course of the next year, they became our best buddies at Charlotte. The four of us would get together and compare our relative experiences with the disease and "the study."

When you are in a situation like we were and you have a chance to talk to someone else in the same situation, your conversation takes on an entirely different tone than when you talk with someone who is not in that same boat. Because of the mutual and genuine understanding of what each other is experiencing, you connect on a different level. You can say and react to things in ways you wouldn't dare with someone else. Mark told us the story of an incident that happened to him early in the disease. His first symptom was weakness in his large muscle groups, so he began experiencing diminished capacity in his arms and legs. One day he had put something away in the attic and was coming down the folding stairs which are located in his garage. He got to the third rung from the bottom and did what he had done all his life: he jumped the rest of the way down. Lying there on the floor, looking up at the ceiling, he said to himself, "Oh yeah. I've got ALS…probably shouldn't jump like that anymore."

The whole time he was recounting this story, he kept shaking his head as if to say, "What a dumb-butt." Well, we were absolutely rolling in the floor with laughter and Marion was right there with us. If you had told me a year earlier that I would be laughing at a guy with ALS who had fallen down, I would have been offended that you could think I was so callous, but it wasn't that way at all. We were simply sharing what we had in common, appreciating the fact someone else knew what we were going through.

Date: Mon 23 Nov 1998 14:21

Hi again,
I took a short nap—about an hour—and felt great. No headache. So I'm running around washing clothes. Decided not to take anything right now to see if it was gone, but now I feel it creeping around my eyebrows so I'll hit the Ibuprofen. I took it at 6am and Tylenol at 10am and that seemed to be the ticket. Anyway I'm tired of the couch so I'm gonna try not to stay there too much.

Sara called around noon to check on me and tell me she wouldn't be home for lunch. I didn't answer the call—it was on her line, but I thought that was sweet of her.

'Nuff said. I love you. Don't feel you need to race home to care for me. I'll be fine and if I'm not, I'll get 'ahold of you.

Love,
Dink

It's Monday. On the previous Friday she had a major operation, during which a bunch of mechanical "stuff" was put into her body and spinal fluid was taken out. She's hobbling around because the incision on her side makes it painful to walk and she's had a headache for seventy–two hours. So, what does she tell me? "Don't worry. I'm fine."

I've never had more admiration.

Date: Tue 24 Nov 1998 10:12

Back again,
Slept from 7:30 until 9:00. I had been reading and dosed off. I'm up now, h/a about 3. Just took some aspirin and more water. I'm dressed neatly, curled my hair. Haven't brushed my teeth yet or done the makeup thing. Brushing kinda bangs my head—if you know what I mean. I found chewing does the same thing.

Anyway, when I woke up, my mind was going 90 to nothing so I have been scribbling ideas on computer sheets. You may think some are cool and others are nuts, but I'm writing them down.

Would you think about talking to Todd Shambo tomorrow about disability for me and more life insurance for me. We really need to get on this before the "boat sails."

I feel another yard sale coming on. A really big one. Get rid of some of this stuff we never use or don't really need. Let the kids mark things they want this Thursday, and we'll keep those things, but clean out and trim down. Use the money to do what we need to for our best interest or our best mental health.

Okay—are you overwhelmed? That was some nap I took, huh?!? I'd make you "tired in the head" if you were here. Of course I would burn up my Lightwriter in the process. I'll let your eyes rest now. Of course if I have gotten you thinking, write your ideas down, too!

I love you,
High Gear Gertie (Dink)

"h/a about 3" On a scale of one–to–ten, her headache was around "three."

Dink had always been plagued by the "early morning busy brains." On those mornings she awoke with her mind racing like that, she could solve all of the world's problems before I was even awake. She would come up with so many things that needed to be done, she could have kept an army busy for a month. On the other side of the bed, I wake up totally stupid…pleasant enough, but completely brain-dead. Many times I would awake to a barrage of questions to which I could only reply, "Baby, can I wake up first or do you HAVE to have an answer right now?"

The Lightwriter was her communication device that could speak what she typed. It was an absolute lifesaver in the way it allowed us to stay connected throughout the disease. At $4500, though, it wasn't something we could just write a check for. In May of '98 we were battling with the insurance company because they said it was not a medical necessity—to which I replied, "Oh yeah? Well, let me put HER on the phone with you, THEN tell me how unnecessary it is!"—when I got a call from the head of the medical staff at NGH. He told me the staff had decided to help us get the Lightwriter and he asked if I would send him some information about it.

We were so touched. Maybe with the money we had put back and some more Dink's parents had sent us, the contribution from the medical staff might allow us to go ahead and get the Lightwriter without having to do more battle with the insurance company.

The next morning Dink dropped off a brochure with the doctor's secretary and that afternoon she got a call asking her to drop by his office to get it back. When she got there, she was handed a check that covered the entire Lightwriter purchase, including accessories and even the shipping costs. We just cried all night. I will never be able to adequately express our gratitude.

Date: Fri 27 Nov 1998 06:39

I LIKE THE SOFTER COLOR ON THE SCREEN. THANKS.

FRIDAYFRIDAYFRIDAYFRIDAYFRIDAYFRIDAYFRIDAYFRIDAY!!!

HAVE A GOOD ONE AND I'LL SEE YOU THIS AFTERNOON. SHORT NOTE- BATHROOM CALLS AND YOU KNOW WHAT THAT IS ALL ABOUT.

LUBS,
DINK

The weakness in her left arm and hand was making it difficult to type so she began using all caps to avoid having to hit the shift key at the beginning of each sentence. It was one of those things she never mentioned. She simply made the needed adjustment and kept moving on.

DECEMBER 1998

Our Family "Tree-dition"

Date: Tue 01 Dec 1998 07:02

Hey sweet thang!
It's 6:50 and I'm ready to go to work, but I just had to send a "honey message" to my pooh bear.

Sara's radio is blasting but I dare not touch it for fear of the wrath of the princess. I find that if we both told her the same thing, she would growl at me and smile at you so I am awarding you the title of Grand Sara Communicator.

I am going to talk with Kathy G. today to tell her about the overtime in Medical Records and work out a way that by the end of the week when the overtime hits the clock I won't be on Nursing II time. I don't want this to hurt her budget any.

I think the Christmas shopping bug has hit me. We need to assess the stash—it isn't as good as last year, but it's something. And it looks like the 70 degree weather may hold on through Christmas so we need to change your mind about no tree while it's 70 degrees or higher. And we don't have to get a huge tree this year unless everyone votes differently.

Well enough blab. Gotta go and you need to get to work, or at least to that 3rd cup of coffee. Have a hugely wonderful day and know that I can't wait to have you in my arms again.

Non-creative end,
Dink

The gift shop at NGH carries some really neat merchandise. As an employee, Dink could make purchases on a payroll deduction plan, so she would always load up during their sales. When Christmas rolled around, we would go through the year's purchases and decide who would get what. Needless to say, a lot of the items, particularly decorations, would end up in our house, but most years she was able to take care of a lot of our Christmas shopping this way.

We've always had a live Christmas tree, even the years we were together before we married. We would load up the whole family and go to a tree farm to cut whichever tree the kids decided was perfect. This yearly trip came to be known as our "family TREE-dition" and it even included getting lost on the way to the tree farm each year. As the kids got older and bigger, we would let them take turns with the handsaw as we cut the tree. It became a privilege of sorts to be the one to have the tree fall on him after making the final cut. Even after Joe and Sara had gone away to college, Sam would insist on making the last cut and wouldn't get up off the ground until I made sure the tree had fallen on top of him. Our favorite years were those marked by cold weather so when we returned home with the tree we could warm up to a big fire and drink hot chocolate. For some reason, it just wasn't the same when we could go tree hunting in shorts and t-shirts, so Dink was softening me up, making sure we wouldn't end up treeless when the kids got out of school for Christmas break.

Date: Tue 08 Dec 1998 07:04

Slept like a big rock last night. Thanks so much for your help. You always come through!

I have ACLS this afternoon so I'm running around getting stuff. I should be home by 5:00, although I am going to try to get groceries again.

I love you,
Dink

Dink worked at NGH for over ten years, serving in a wide variety of nursing positions, from floor nurse to charge nurse to department manager. She worked as Patient and Staff Education Coordinator for a couple of years, which involved a good bit of actual instruction time. We talked often about the fact we were both teachers while she was in that position. She eventually became certified as an instructor in numerous varieties of CPR, including Advanced Cardiac Life Support (ACLS). By December of '98, she was totally dependent on the Lightwriter for communication, but she was still teaching effectively. She managed to do so by developing a series of media-based instructional units to present her lesson content, which allowed her to concentrate on student evaluation. That approach resulted in a successful learning environment for her students that was void of lecture. I know a lot of professional educators who would shudder at the thought.

JANUARY 1999

Sorry, Papa John

From: DinkC
To: BevE, et al
Subject: Dink's 1998 Reflections for Family and Friends
Date: Fri 1 Jan 1999 09:37

I am sitting here reflecting on 1998. Sadness, frustration, sure. But the emotion that best describes it all is pure joy.

I have reunited with my brother, Redding, and his "girls." I have reunited with my soul-cousin, Ken Christian and his family. My parents and my brother and sisters and I celebrated my parents' 50th wedding anniversary with 160+ friends. Bennie and Sybil Gandy: 4 children, 11 grandchildren. No great-grands yet and I don't see any chance for the near future. We're just trying to get Chuck, Joe, Hank, and Rebecca out of college, Sara into and out of post-grad school, and all of them joining the work force so they can pay their own car insurance.

My other set of parents, Clyde and Myrtis Hobby, also celebrated their 50th wedding anniversary this year. They went on a "to die for" cruise in the Mediterranean. Awhhhhhhhhhh! They didn't have room in their suitcase for me. Myrtis and Clyde Hobby: 2 children, 6 grandchildren. Again, none close to great grands (see Joe, Sara, and Rebecca, above)

How blessed I am to have two such wonderful examples of strong, enduring marriages to lead me through my own marriage. Praise God and His creations!

My somber ALS neurologist at Emory got lured to Charlotte, North Carolina, to set up a wonderful ALS clinic where I get a complete evaluation while I visit with other *PALS* (People with ALS) and Alan gets to visit also—so we don't feel so all alone with our "ALS project." And my doctor is no longer somber—he's in his element—laughing, visiting, and now immersed, thankfully for me and so many others, in research looking for a cure.

I saw the doctors at the hospital where I have worked for ten years, in a humbling action, buy my communication aide! I was floored! Alan and I cried for joy and in humble thanksgiving. It came at just the right time. My speech was moving from slurred to s-l-u-r-r-e-d. Now less than 5% of what I say is understandable to Alan and the kids. But, I am typing at the speed of light with my little communicator. And the kids gave me a speaker phone for Christmas so I can communicate in one more way. Wonderful!

Okay, Snippets:

Sara—23 years old—graduated from the University of Georgia and moved back home to make some money and contemplate her future. Her major: exercise science. She is working for an ophthalmologist, babysitting for the high society moms, and working in Athens at Athens Regional Hospital in the physical therapy department. Sara the whirlwind!

Joseph—21 years old—graduated from boot camp—yes we traipsed to Fort "Lost in the Woods," Missouri, in the middle of winter. Three days later and we would have gotten snowed in. But Joe graduated then headed to individual training (A.I.T.) and graduated two days after his 21st birthday. He spent his birthday in a tent, in the mud. He has been working in Athens and will be heading back to school in January. He's in the Army Reserve. He also continues his pursuits to form the perfect band.

Sam is fifteen. 'Nuff' said. Not really. He is a sophomore at Newton High. His grades are wonderful. He studies without being told! Wow! He is very active in our church youth program and is becoming a leader there. He helps with Childrens' Church, has been drafted to teach a few younger-aged classes and is on the missions committee and the committee on committees. His other passion is cars. We have a '77, red Camaro and a '71, electric blue Torino. As soon as he has money, another part for one of the cars. He turns 16 in March.

Alan teaches DCT (work-study) at Eagles Landing High School in Henry County. He hit a deer this year on the way to school (in Joe's car.) Really messed up the car—good thing Joe was in Missouri. His mother is going to be moving up here in the spring, or thereabout. We've been looking around at places to show her. He has been a real champ, going with me for every doctor visit. Driving the 5 hours up and 5 hours back going to Charlotte to the ALS clinic.

I am still working at Newton General Hospital. I audit charts for documentation problems. I work in Utilization Review in peak times and in Medical Records changing the diseases into numbers so the insurance companies can figure them out. I have found out there is a lot of work there for someone with a brain but no speech. I am busier now than when I worked on the unit. Oh, I still get called to put in IVs and help with information or a hug when things are crazy.

So, my 1998 was a busy year. So many changes. So many challenges. So many opportunities. I hope 1999 provides the same. May God bless each of you with peace, joy, and the comfort of knowing He is in control, so don't sweat the small stuff.

I love you all. We love you all. Happy New Year.

Alan, Debra, Sara, Joe, & Sam
Coleman

Dink had never written one of these "This Was Our Year" letters. In fact, although we did enjoy reading the ones we received each year in our Christmas Cards, we always thought they were kinda cheesy. Now, if you're a dedicated "This Was Our Year" writer, please don't take offense. We just never imagined anyone being that interested in our family history. But this year was different. When you're dealing with something as huge as a terminal disease, everyone seems to want to know how you're doing.

Reading over this message again just now, it occurred to me that she didn't say a whole lot about what we did in 1998. And, except for her speech, she didn't mention her physical condition. Instead, she talked mostly about the people she loved, from whom she drew so much of the strength she needed to make it through the disease. I can't imagine how we would have coped without this circle of love.

Date: Tue 19 Jan 1999 07:31

Hey my great car driver,
Mom called. She is putting the bag in overnight delivery so no Cracker Barrel for you my dear.

See you tonight. Drive safely and always know.....

YOU DA ONE, BABEE!

I love to eat at Cracker Barrel. If I ate there as much as I would like, I would BECOME a barrel. Dink had left a bag she needed at her parent's house after a weekend visit. Our original plan to get it back involved meeting her folks for supper at the Cracker Barrel in Macon, which is about half way between our two homes. Not to worry, there were plenty more opportunities for me to work on my "barrelness."

Date: Wed 20 Jan 1999 06:42

Mornin' babee,
Stirring kinda slow today, but what else is new? You looked exceptionally sharp in that yellow and blue! Yum!

Thanks for getting Sam today. I think I will put in a few extra hours and try to make up for being out on Monday.

Have a great day and know, somebunny lubs ya!

Forever and even now,
Dink

Date: Fri 22 Jan 1999 06:59

Hey!
I finally got that pie almost fixed. It's 6:44 and it's chilling for 2 minutes then to the crust I made last night. I had a time with the blue and green food coloring. The coloring I bought yesterday didn't say gel decorating stuff, it just said food coloring. I admit I didn't read the directions to see if you have to dissolve it in hot water, but I'm kinda dense in the morn-

ings these days—I think it's those flannel sheets and my snuggy pal. Deep snoozin'.

I'm sending a note to Bobbie Dooley along with this one to you.

I just poured filling into crust. Crust too small, had a major overrun, so we can eat lime chiffon pie and I'll throw a cake on this afternoon—or we'll hit a deli. I should stop trying those new recipes for events.

Well I'm bummed! Gonna go get in the shower and try not to be late to work. Have a terrific day and come home to me safe and sound. If you get home before me, start that cake—the box is in the pantry. Chocolate cake with white icing. If you just want to get it mixed, I'll get it in the pans and bake then ice.

I'm going to try to be home by 4:30. See you then.

Snow as a slail,   _____ as a _____
Dink

Bobbie Dooley is an ALS patient we never met face-to-face. In fact, I don't remember exactly how we came to know of her, but she and Dink became big email buds. Total strangers becoming close, valued, personal friends because of shared circumstances…we saw it happen so many times and that synergy was absolutely vital to our daily emotional strength. We simply could not have survived the disease without it.

Dink was an excellent cook, but she was notorious for trying a new recipe when we had plans that involved her cooking for other people. Sometimes they worked great…sometimes we ended up taking pizza.

Date: Wed 27 Jan 1999 07:41

Hey lubber boy!
Didn't get your email last night in time. But it was nice just to vege out
and head to bed early.

I can't decide if I am hot or cold this morning. Ambiguous weather! I've
got a Clint Black song that really sounds like you and something you
have strong feelings regarding. I'll share that with you when we get a
chance.

We have a dinner/pot luck date with Larry and Catherine Parnell at
their house not this one but next weekend. The day and menu aren't
fixed yet. I thought you might enjoy a quiet, hilarious evening with
friends.

Well, gotta go. Have a fab' day. Come home and give me a great big
Bear-Al hug this afternoon, and my thoughts of you will be happy-
packed all day.

Lubber, slubber,
Dink

*Catherine Parnell is the administrative assistant to the Director of Nursing
Services at NGH and was one of Dink's closest friends. Her husband Larry
also works at NGH in the security division. They are an absolute hoot. You
simply can't be around them for more than a minute without breaking into
laughter. On top of that, they are one of the most loving and caring couples
I have ever known.*

*I did manage to talk Dink into using one of her tried-and-true recipes for
this dinner. Sorry, Papa John.*

FEBRUARY 1999

Remember to Call

Date: Tue 02 Feb 1999 06:28

Hey sweetie,
I know I stretched twice this morning and that always ends with that loud long exhale. If I continue to wake you up, we need to work on some changes. Maybe with furloughs on the weekend.

Last night, while you were cooking and I was "groupie-ing," there were 2 things needed—dog food and _____—I forgot. If you remember, could you call me? I'm not sure how your day will play out so if this isn't convenient, nix it. I'll get the dog food and the other when I remember.

I hope everything goes great for you and the school today. I hope your day in particular is just amazingly wonderful.

Bub 'n' rubbles,   _____ 'n' _____
Dink

I am a very light sleeper, which is both good and bad. It was good she could wake me easily if she needed something but not so good because she could wake me accidently too, sometimes without even waking herself. It's odd though, because I snore like a freight train yet I rarely wake myself. If she could get to sleep before I started snoring, she could sleep right through it too, but if she awoke during the night and I was already snoring, she could-n't get back to sleep. Anyway, she eventually suggested sleeping in separate rooms so we wouldn't interfere with each others snooze time, which was the sensible thing to do, but neither one of us liked it…so we didn't do it very often.

Date: Thu 04 Feb 1999 06:54

Hey Lubber Boy,
I got an email from Beverly Elder: Feb 19 at 9:00am. Is that good?

A few reminders—
    Call Dr. Leonard
    Call Bulldog Tire Company
    Call me crazy but you're my guy.

I never heard back from Sam about Prayer Breakfast so I guess my help-ing with transportation would be too great an embarrassment for a nearly 16 kinda kid.

I should have worked on that article last night and finished it but it did-n't even cross my mind—even when looking straight at it! Talking about un-focused! But that cake is going to be killer!

I need to talk with Catherine Parnell this day and find out which evening we are getting together—Friday or Saturday. I think we just left it to this weekend.

I'd better go. Things to do, places to drive to, make a baby coo…the list is endless. You have a most amazing day and bring yourself back to my arms this evening. And……REMEMBER TO CALL.

Magging Nomma,
Dink

Bev Elder was the original study coordinator for the BDNF study. She was terrific…very loving and incredibly easy to get along with. We would go in for an appointment that should last thirty minutes and it would take two hours because we would end up visiting with Bev for so long.

Dink had offered to provide weekly transportation from Prayer Breakfast to school for Sam and any others that needed it. He was within two months of getting his driver's license, so I don't think there was any way he was going to let Mama take him to school.

Date: Fri 05 Feb 1999 08:03

DR. LEONARD DR. LEONARD DR. LEONARD

CALLCALLCALLCALLCALLCALLCALLCALL

WHOLEWEEKWASTEDWHOLEWEEKWASTED

LOVELOVELOVELOVELOVELOVELOVE

Dink

Dr. Carolyn Leonard is our dentist and is married to Dr. Leon Leonard, the kid's orthodontist. During the time the kids had mouths full of metal, we differentiated between the two doctors by saying "Dr. Mr. Leonard" or "Dr.

Ms. Leonard." Between all five of us seeing her and two of the kids seeing him, my guess would be we personally financed about ten percent of the huge new home they built a few years ago.

Date: Tue 09 Feb 1999 05:19

Hey babee,
Just woke up and heard you getting up and then felt my bladder talking. When I got up and you were in your robe, it threw me a little. Anyway, after the bathroom trip, I couldn't get back to sleep and I didn't realize it was 3am. But I had a wonderful hot bath and washed my hair and I'll get to work early.

Have a great day today. Are there any cars to fix today? I've lost count.

Love forevermore,
Dink

We had six cars in the family and the newest was a '93 Chevy, so it seemed like we were always repairing one. Bless her heart, Sara began referring to our yard as a used car lot.

Date: Fri 12 Feb 1999 06:47

Mornin' gloree,
I knew I was getting loud last night so I went ahead and got up. I lay down on the couch and my hip just wouldn't settle down. So, I decided to get up and take a bath and get ready for work and I walked to the kitchen to check the time. 1:42!!!!—that's real misery. I pondered and pondered what to do because my book was in the room with you, and I didn't want to start an active project that would wake me up for the

duration. I decided to switch my head to the other end of the couch. High tech answers in a high tech world.

So I finally settled in. Next thing I know, you're leaving. I know we don't bond much in the morning but not to get a skin hug? 1:42 and no good hug? My Friday can only get better! By the time you get home tonight, I'll be a walking party I suspect.

Have a super dooper day and don't accept no wooden nickels. Remind me to tell you about Troy Brooks. It's a funny story. Bring yourself home to me tonight—I'll be pondering on that very thing today.

Hunnin' fy tingers rhru mour yair,

_____ _____ _____ _____ _____ _____

Dink

Date: Fri 12 Feb 1999 19:19
Subject: Re: How-DEE

How come this email got to me seven days late? Was it on the 1st, 2nd or 3rd list?

Lubs back to you,
Dink

On Fri, 05 Feb 1999 04:05:12 PST
"Alan Coleman" writes:

Hey Sweetie-Boom,
Just wanted to shoot one at ya to say "hope the faxing went well" and that you have a wondermous day. See ya this eve'. I love you.   AC

I think this is the only time she wrote to me by replying to a message I had sent to her.

Date: Tue 16 Feb 1999 06:34

You are the absolute best!!! Thank you for all the work you did yesterday and for being such a good dad. You're amazing!—and I'm so blessed to have you with me.

Have a tremendous day and bring that ＿＿＿ body back to me this evening- I need my hug!

Love to the googley—ith degree,
Dink

I'm not a journal keeper, but sometimes I wish I was: I have absolutely no clue what we did on Monday, February 15, 1999.

MARCH 1999

The Significance of Adoption

Date: Mon 01 Mar 1999 13:07
Subject: news and reminders

Hey my stud muffin,
I ran home for lunch so I'm sending you a few things.

I paged you this AM for your mom, she didn't know if you had the lot number—about 7:35am. When I got into the car, as I was driving I heard a noise and lo and behold—there was your pager. It has our page and a voice mail before ours. I forget day and time and I'm too lazy to limp out to the car for it.

Don't forget to make an appt. with Todd Shambo about disability. I was thinking—we could also put extra into my retirement acct. That would help, too.

Nothing else to report. Your mom has been cleaning dishes. I've been putting them up. She's got Estelle's room number at Kennestone Hospital.

Well that's all. I may pick Sam up after school then go back in for a few hours. Maybe I can tolerate split up days better.

I love you. Need to stop and eat. Left over pizza. I think your mom may be stir crazy. Ok, I'll stop.

Lubs and lore mubs, _____ and _____ _____
Dink

Date: Mon 01 Mar 1999 16:33

Hey again,
2 numbers on pager: 770xyz9339 and 770xyz2084

See ya soon. EsteMom's waited all day and now at 4:00 she thinks Harriet won't call. You might want to give your mom a call.

Lubs—I picked Sam up from school and had lunch with EsteMom (she's watching her soap right now), so the only one I haven't given attention to is you. I think that would be a mutual benefit.

I'm headed back to work. I'll work until I get tired again. I think ya'll can fend for supper. I want you to think about visiting Joe next Tuesday. Call first, but I think ya'll would have a great time talking.

Well, enough!
Dink

My mother was in the process of moving to our area from South Georgia and was staying with us a few days to take care of some real estate details. She is the only person I have ever known whose name is Estelene. She was adamant for years that she would not be called Granny or Grandma or anything of that nature, so when her first grandchild was born she insisted

on the name EsteMom. Recently I set up an email account for her and
threatened to start calling her "E-mom."

Date: Fri 05 Mar 1999 05:45

My sleepy fellow,
Sorry for the awful 3am to 5am. I thought I saw the windows lightened
so I thought it was close to 5. Then I got up and it was 3 and I knew I
was Screwed.

I hope Friday is sweet to you. This weekend is going to be so busy! Life
races on.

You have been so wonderful for and to me. It's amazing how far we have
come. All things to God's purpose.

Sweepless aights and sleet nfternoon saps,
_____ _____ *and* _____ _____ _____
Dink

We had a really rough time in our marriage in the early part of the 1990's.
There were times we could have killed each other and occasionally we
tried—not literally, but emotionally. We never spoke of actually ending
the marriage, though, because we were each too stubborn and prideful to
end up having to say we failed at it. Because we were so committed to
making it work, we eventually set aside our anger at each other and got
back to doing what we had done the night we met. We started talk-
ing...and talking...and talking. I'm not even sure when we reached the
point that our marriage was no longer in trouble, but even after we got
there, we kept talking and talking. I'm not yet certain how much of our
lives are specifically directed by God, but I'm convinced He allowed us to

experience that troubled time in our marriage so we could develop the strength and resolve we would need as a couple to successfully face the disease.

Date: Tue 09 Mar 1999 06:51

Hey babee!
How's it shakin'? I feel wonderful this morning! My arm still hurts but my hips are so much better and my shoulders don't burn like they did. Thank you so much for putting action to my idea. You complete the team of Dink-n-Al quite well! Kudos!

This is a short one. Egg on stove for Sam, need to make a list of the stuff I woke up thinking, etc, etc...

Snoves, luggles, and snibbles,   _____ _____ and _____
Dink

ALS is such a perplexing disease. In and of itself, the disease causes no pain, yet she was constantly experiencing some in a variety of places in her body. We had reasoned that some of it might be caused by her relative level of inactivity, while some of it was probably caused by adjustments she had to make to compensate for weakening muscles. Those adjustments involved non-natural movements which would cause strain on muscles that might not even be involved in the disease yet. She came up with some in-home physical therapy ideas we tried and had some success with, and I got to be her physical therapist. That was a neat turn-about. In 1989, I had shoulder surgery and I remember how she had way too much fun being my "physical terrorist" back then. It was payback time.

Date: Tue 09 Mar 1999 13:21

Guess what I found in the hood of my jacket a few minutes ago——a chicken nugget!

Home for lunch and going back to resume coding. I'll see you this drizzly afternoon. Let's cuddle up in front of the fire with all the lights out. Except for the fire and a few candles.

I pick up my wrist and ankle braces Thursday at 2:45.
From drippy,
Dink

One of the ongoing topics of discussion in our marriage was the fact she was not the most organized, systematic, or neat person in the world, which had humorous implications in the discovery of a chicken nugget in the hood of her jacket.

The weaknesses on her left side that began appearing in October had become more involved. Her left foot had developed a condition called "foot drop." She could no longer flex her foot upward, so she was having to limp in order to walk without tripping on her toe. Her left hand was basically limp and, without correction, would curl up toward the underside of her wrist. The braces helped her offset these problems…to a limited extent…as the bionic conversion continued.

Date: Wed 10 Mar 1999 06:45

Hey babe,
Did you hear Spiff's "God Bless America" about 6:45? About one town's fight against the moving stereo blasters the teens use. I had to sit down I was laughing so hard!

Anyway, hope the day is great. Not sure about time for me. If I'm hurting I'll be home well before 5. If not, I'll make a conscious effort to "get to the church on time."

Slubs and ricky,   _____ *and* _____
Dink

Spiff is one of the morning deejays at a local radio station. Very funny guy.

We have Wednesday Night Supper at our church each week and she was notorious for getting there about the time they stopped serving. I don't specifically remember if she made it on time that night or not.

Date: Wed 10 Mar 1999 10:56

Hey sweetie,
Read your nugget reply—you're sooo cute!

Well I knew I was in trouble the second time I had to sit down this morning. I got to work at 7:30 and by 9:00 I couldn't take just sitting. My hips and upper legs ache and I feel like I need to move—restless legs.

Anyway, at home I can go at my own pace and get a few things done. If you get a chance, slide on home prior to 4:00 and we'll slide dance. That don't hurt none.

See ya' later, studerater,
Dink

Another perplexing aspect of ALS is hyperactivity. The universal character-
istic of the disease is that it causes a person to lose the use of their muscles,
but in the process of doing that, it causes those same muscles to be hyperac-
tive. Often times, she could not sit comfortably because her legs would
twitch so much. In fact, they would wake her up at night if we didn't get
her propped just right. It was so frustrating. I can remember us looking at
each other and thinking, "What the heck is that all about!?!"

Date: Thu 11 Mar 1999 13:52
Subject: Re: "Nooner" e-words

I love it when you "nooner" me.

I'd love a date with my fine sexy hunk of sweetness. I didn't make it to
work. Shoulders and hips were hurting and I couldn't sit very long,
soooo-

I went to the church to do the sign. I needed to run it past Len and
Bobby. After Bobby left, Len started talking about a dear friend of his
who had died with ALS. And about his friend that's near death now. The
nerve! I cried through 3/4's of a box of Kleenex. I told him about Alan
Hobby dying on me and how I empathize a bit deeply with those left
behind. I also told him about your wondrous rescue. Even before I said
all that, he had said that you are quite a guy! He really likes you. Can you
see my tears?

Okay. Back to dryness. What do you want to see tonight? Syrup or comedy or drama or adventure or suspense or..................I look forward
to it with great expectations.

Love divided by two is one,
DinkAL

Sometimes I would email her at lunchtime…a "nooner."

Dink was on the Evangelism Committee at church and had volunteered to do the weekly messages on the marquee sign in front of the building. Len Strozier is our pastor and Bobby Sims is our music minister and I guess she wanted to get their approval on the new sign message.

Alan Hobby was Dink's high school sweetheart and first husband. He was a young, strong, healthy farmer who had a bad bout with influenza in November of 1977, then died of congestive heart failure in June of the next year. Dink explained that the flu spread down around his heart and made it weak. Nothing could have prevented it. She was twenty–two years old and was left with two kids under the age of three. She and the kids moved to Athens in 1980 so she could attend the Medical College of Georgia, School of Nursing to get her bachelors degree. They moved in across the hall from my apartment and, even before I met her, I started playing with Sara and Joe when I would see them out in the yard. After we got to know each other and started hanging out together, I would baby-sit the kids when she had to work. We worked out a deal where I wouldn't charge her any money, but I would have free reign in her kitchen. That worked out pretty good except the time I ate a whole bag of chocolate chip cookies and she didn't find out until she had already poured a glass of milk for Joe and went to the pantry to get the cookies she had just promised him. I payed penance that evening by buying four bags of chocolate chip cookies…one for each of us. I still got the best end of our arrangement, though, because it would have been a lot cheaper for her to hire someone else than it was to keep me fed.

After we got married I adopted Sara and Joe. We always thought it was cool that she and Alan Hobby had given Joe the middle name Alan, because Alan is my middle name also. When Sam was born, we couldn't resist: Samuel Alan Coleman.

My entire impression of adoption changed when I adopted Joe and Sara. I had always heard the significance of being adopted was that your parents had "chosen" you to adopt. To me though, the significance of adoption is its total completeness. When I adopted The Bigs (Joe and Sara's collective nick-name), the State of Georgia issued new birth certificates for them listing me as their biological father. From a legal standpoint, it's as if it had never been any other way. Joe and Sara are MY kids, plain and simple. Isn't that awesome?

Date: Tue 16 Mar 1999 13:21

Hey my sleepy head,
I have been rescued from tomorrow's 2 hr. baby sitting. I lasted only 3 hours at work. I stood up to code. Finally I faxed Dr. Stillerman about the pain and then 45 min. later, I went over to his office. He thinks I'm right on the money regarding my limp causing the pain. I am scheduled for a cat scan and myelogram tomorrow at 10:30. I am hoping you can take this time off. I will be in observation until the afternoon. I have paged you and I hope either that or this gets your attention.

Bubs and lainful putts,   _____ and _____ _____
Dink

One of Dink's responsibilities at the hospital was chart coding. Apparently every procedure performed in a hospital has a universally recognized code assigned to it. After a patient leaves the hospital, his chart is sent to the Medical Records department where it is reviewed and all of the appropriate codes are added. It's typically a desk job, but between her pain and her twitching legs, she often had to stand up to do it.

While Dink was home during this period of time, she sent several faxes to Catherine Parnell. As I include them, they will be preceded by "From: Alan & Debra Coleman Home Fax."

From: Alan & Debra Coleman Home Fax
To: Catherine Parnell
03/17/99

Mornin' Sunshine,
CT and myelogram changing to MRI per ALS team. Something about the preservative in the myelogram dye and the material in my catheter. The MRI is okay with my titanium implant, although it will stop the pump and erase the memory. Now not to worry (here's why I go to Charlotte to my beloved team). When they got my 2:00pm email regarding the ct/myelo, they got on the phone to the pump company headquarters and to the drug people at headquarters, arranged for my pump rep to be at the hospital with me to instantly reprogram my pump when the MRI is over, and emailed me back with an emergency "plans need to change"...including my nurse's home phone number so we could discuss and plan from my end. If Sidney, the pump rep, has time, I'll introduce her to you and Barbara and Kathy and Mr. Weadick. How's that!

Hove and Lugs to All   _____ *and* _____ *to All*
Debra C.

Date: Wed 17 Mar 1999 14:09

ALAN,
        I NEED TO SPEAK WITH YOU RIGHT NOW.
Dink

Dink was scheduled to have some tests done at NGH, but the plans changed, resulting in our needing to go to the medical center in another county. The urgency in the email above is explained in the following fax message.

From: Alan & Debra Coleman Home Fax
To: Catherine Parnell
03/17/99

I'm sorry Catherine,
Sidney is stuck in Charlotte and the local rep is in Macon with another pump implant, so I have to go to Dekalb Medical Center to get reprogrammed. Shoot!

Till Later,
DEBRA C.

I did call her within a few minutes of her sending that urgent sounding email so she could tell me about the change in plans. She went ahead and had the MRI at Newton General, then we hurried forty-five minutes to the Dekalb County Medical Center to have her pump reprogrammed. We actually saw a cancer specialist for the reprogramming. Many of his patients used a pump similar to Dink's for administering pain medication. Beginning early in the disease, we said many times we were grateful that the disease Dink had was not a pain intensive disease like cancer. After visiting a doctor who used "the pump" for pain relief purposes we reaffirmed that gratitude.

Date: Mon 22 Mar 1999 14:01

Hey my sweet babee,
How is the day going? Much improvement here. I got up about 9:00 and showered and took my usual meds but no Darvocet or Flexeril. I am still

a little foggy from them and I don't think it's wise for me to be driving. Tomorrow afternoon I need to go in and do my mandatory education recert. I also need to go in from 8:00—12:00 on Thursday. I might be able to do the mandatory ed on Thursday too. I'll have to check on check-off times.

Well, your mom and I had a huge laugh this morning. She was getting ready to take some stuff to her house and she said, "Well I'm pretty sure I have things together."

To which I replied, "No!" We rolled for 15 minutes, it was great!

She called John Crudson's office this morning and she wants you to help her call the builders—we couldn't find their number.

That's it from home. I'm tackling the ironing today. Such fun! But it's a labor of love. I love you so very much, I'll even iron for you—occasionally. Until I see you this afternoon…….

Geepy and sloofy,   _____ *and* _____
Dink

My dear mother has a long history of leaving things behind. Through the years when she would come to visit us, after she left to go back home, we would search through the house looking for whatever she had forgotten. We always found something. We even designated a spot in one closet for the "EsteMom Stuff."

Date: Thu 25 Mar 1999 11:09

Hey sweet thang',
Hope thing's are going well for you this dreary day. I have the alcohol for the rear view mirror if you want to come by here before ya'll go to the test.

Sam was really bummed this morning. We got started 5 minutes late and we needed to go by the instant banker. Well we got to Stone Road and the car started making a funny sound. The air conditioner hose had a big rip in it so we came back home but we couldn't find the duct tape I gave you to put up the other day. Great job of putting it up but can you share its location with us?

I got groceries after I dropped him off at Chic Filet. I got a 35 lb. bag of dog food that really tried to whip me. You should have seen me dragging it around! What a sight.

The back pain is better each day. I think by Monday I will be able to sit comfortably. But if not, I have over 200 extended illness hours that are lost when you leave NGH. I sure am proud of the cleaning and sorting we are doing. I even bought ammonia so I can strip all those layers of wax off the kitchen floor.

Well, let me go. Things to do. Be careful driving home if it is raining. I am praying for a 2 hour window without rain from 2 until 4. I just don't want to face Sam if this doesn't work out today. I'll see you later. Wrap yourself in my cozy love quilt.

Snugs and heezes,　　　　　　　_____ and _____
Dink

Sam's sixteenth birthday was on Sunday, March 21, 1999. When Sam turned fifteen, he had to wait a couple days to get his learner's license because the license office was closed on his birthday. In Georgia, you have to have your learner's permit for a full year before you can get your driver's permit, so he couldn't get the latter on his sixteenth birthday, even if it had not been on Sunday. At 16 years and four days old, he was finally qualified to get his license but we woke up to rain and the license office won't do driver testing on wet roads. Poor kid had to wait another day.

Date: Fri 26 Mar 1999 12:03

What a bee-you-tee-full day! Sam must be sitting on pins and needles. Before you take him to the office, go around the square and tell him how to handle the signs and yields. I know he will be terrific!

Well I want to get out and play in the dirt.

Fubs 4 lever, _____ _____
Dink

The boy turned his frown upside-down that afternoon.

Date: Mon 29 Mar 1999 06:39
Subject: COMPUTER VIRUS WARNING!!!!! OPEN FIRST!!!!!!

Hey babee,
First of all! I heard on the radio that a computer virus is spreading through email and it starts with, "an important message from......" It was reported on Fox News and it isn't April Fool's Day today so I take it to be truthful. So beware when you jump on your email.

I got up right after you left. I think I'll concentrate on our bedroom and bathroom today. If time and exhaustion allow, I really need to strip the kitchen floor. I'll need a few hours when ya'll aren't here so I can air out the ammonia smell before ya'll come home.

Two of my irises in the front yard have shot up stems with the promise of multiple beautiful white blossoms. I love spring—and summer and fall and winter. Each carries its own mysteries and surprises. Kinda like you. This…..I love.

Will you go by Mike Brown's on your way home and pick up those banners and thank him profusely for his generous gift. Then this afternoon, we need to get those put up and change the big sign in front at the church.

Well, be careful driving today and I hope you have a simply extraordinarily wonderful day. Til then…..

Snold moes and corning tuggles,

_____ _____ *and* _____ _____

Dink

Mike Brown is a local sign maker and a member of our church. He donated a couple of large banners to advertise an upcoming Spring Revival at the church. When I got to his shop he wasn't there, but as I came through town I noticed he had already put the banners up himself. Thanks again, Mike.

She spoke of her fondness for all of the seasons, but Spring was her favorite by far. She loved to "play in the dirt" then anxiously await the colors that would eventually pop up. Before she got sick she would go to a local nursery and come back with a trunk load of flowers and bulbs and peat moss and anything else that had caught her eye. When I would ask about her planting plan she would say, "I have no idea. I just thought they were pretty." She would plant, they would bloom, and it always turned out beautifully.

Obviously we didn't know it at the time, but she wrote this on the first day of the last year of her life. I find it strangely ironic that she mentioned all four seasons—one year—then experienced each one only one more time.

APRIL 1999

Now I'm Crying!! Blast!!

From: Alan & Debra Coleman Home Fax
To: Catherine Parnell
April 01, 1999

MORNIN' CAT-WOMAN,
I think the up and down from yesterday backfired. I woke up at around 4:30 with fire in my back and both upper legs. That hasn't happened in two days. And the pain hasn't been that bad for several more days. So I will probably just wait until Alan gets home this afternoon, then come in to do a little work on the cancer report to the state. I can stand to do most of that, or if I have to sit, I won't have to sit long.

It was soooooo very great to see everyone yesterday. It's like a tonic. Hug therapy is the greatest. And I passed the test. I even hugged Greg Richardson, who did the sexual harassment speech in mandatory ed. So I guess I'll get those towels folded and run a couple of wash loads and maybe dry them and fold them, too. And I guess I'll mop the kitchen and the bathroom. And I guess I'll…Boy! I'm tired already!

That's my pitiful story for today. I'll have to stop here because my hips are burning. You and Larry are our sweethearts. Give a few hugs for me today.

Bincerely from sain in the putt,
_____ *from* _____ *in the* _____
Debra Coleman

Greg Richardson, Director of Human Resources at NGH, is a very profes-
sional professional...a VERY professional professional. He's friendly
enough when he needs to be, but for the most part he's much more com-
fortable within the defined roles and rules of professional etiquette. He
serves the hospital extremely well in his position because he is very much
"by the book." The whole touchy-feely-huggy thing is pretty much lost on
Greg at work, so it was quite humorous to Dink that she was able to give
him a hug within days of his presenting a class on sexual harassment. I
can't help wondering if she thought about giving him a little pat on the
boot...just to see how he'd react.

Date: Fri 02 Apr 1999 09:18

Hi azalia strong man,
I hope school isn't too difficult for you today. That red shirt should
ward off any evil spirits. I am so touched by your searching for me. I just
can't believe how close we have become. Of course, now I'm crying!!
Blast!! It really is so very special.

I want you to check out a couple of businesses. The first is a disability
insurance, I think, kinda place: http//directory.xyz.com. The other is
http//www.xyz.com/nationalife- I just want to see their requirements.

It's around 8:45 and Sam hasn't stirred. I have started cleaning our
bathroom. It should be spic and span by the time you get home. If I'm
not totally worn out by then I'll start on the kitchen. Nah! That'll be
another day. Right now I have our bathroom trash can and assorted

cleaning brushes running alone in the dishwasher. I hope we can stop the mildew problem. I think we should start drying off the windows after we take a shower, if they are wet.

Well enough gab. I'm stalling! Again, have a great day and I will see your handsome mug this afternoon. Love forever and ever.

Snubs and rooches,   _____ and _____
Dink

P.S. Remind me to tell you about the appendage dream.

We went out in the yard during the previous evening to plan our Spring cleanup and planting, but Dink's walking was getting to the point that it was hard for me to relax when she was out of my reach. Her gait had become so unsteady that I was nervous because I knew she might fall. It was so hard to know what to do in those situations because Dink was so ferociously independent. She didn't want me hovering over her, but I didn't want her to be too far away. After we exchanged some stern looks, she convinced me she was alright on her own, so we started drifting further apart. When I wanted to check on her, I had to sneak a peek because it would make her mad if I watched too closely. Indeed, she did seem to be handling the yard's terrain well enough and had even overcome a momentary loss of balance, so with that reassurance, I headed around the corner of the house.

After inspecting the front yard a few minutes and trying to mentally picture a new planting bed she told me she wanted to build, I realized it had been several minutes since I last checked on her. I stepped right to the corner of the house and attempted to appear to be casually glancing in her direction and there she was sitting on the ground. With a slightly embarrassed look on her face, she raised her arms with her palms facing upward

*and shrugged her shoulders, as if to say, "Gee, I don't know what hap-
pened." Still peering around the corner of the house, I asked, "Fell down?"
and she nodded her head affirmatively. "You OK?" and she nodded her
head again. "Need help?" and she folded her hands at her chin as if to
say "Please." I helped her up and we continued our survey of the yard
but I stayed right by her side the rest of the way. She didn't seem to mind
anymore.*

From: Alan & Debra Coleman Home Fax
To: Catherine Parnell
April 12, 1999

Praise and good tidings my sister,
After 3 days of a total of 8 hours sleep, I finally was exhausted enough to
sleep through the night. I've been catching up on my emails this morning. Dr. Rosenfeld emailed me back yesterday and he's going to put me
on Tegretol for the back and leg pain. Please pray for me and this new
treatment.

Sara called me yesterday and said Medical College of Ga School of
Physical Therapy hadn't made their decisions, yet, so we will have to put
a deposit down on her spot at Ga State in case Med. Coll. falls through.
I think Med. Coll. would be fools to pass over Sara and her extensive
work history in physical therapy, but that's a Mama's opinion. Here's
another area I need your prayers.

I miss all of ya'll and hope I can come back soon. Hold down the fort for
me and you are in my prayers, too.

Love,
Debra C.

Date: Tue 13 Apr 1999 10:21

Mornin'
Life springs anew. I remember you leaving, but I rolled over at 8:30 and finally pulled it together and got up at 9:00. I saw the email from Dr. Rosenfeld, so I guess you will need to go by the hospital today sometime for the Tegretol.

It was so nice not to have such pain while spooning. I was having the usual stinging in my legs when I got in bed, but the full effect of sleeplessness caught up with me when my head hit that pillow. I only remember being awake that one time I got up. I know you got up after me but I don't remember you gettin back in bed. Wow!

Well, let me go. Have a super day. Only 37 more. I'll see you this afternoon.

Cherishingly yours,
Dink

As the wife of a school teacher, Dink had long ago realized the importance of the "End of the Year Countdown." Every teacher does one and if they tell you they don't, they're lying. ;o}

From: Alan & Debra Coleman Home Fax
To: Catherine Parnell
April 13, 1999

Mornin "Aunt Cat,"
Those boys were so angelic looking during their baptism. I am so glad you and Larry were there to share the joy. Will and Taylor were so serious and Austin had that "Wow! Everyone is looking at me!" look. As I

remember last summer's Vacation Bible School, all three boys plus several more were anything but angels. They were part of a group of 24 their age in VBS. When we were getting our pre-VBS assignments, Tracy Croom traded with me so she wouldn't have her own daughter. I had 5 four–to–five–year–olds and poor Tracy ended up with the group of 24. My son, Sam, helped her and every time I saw him he had at least 3 kids hanging onto him.

By the way, how did you like Sam's children's sermon? Len Strozier, our pastor, asked Sam to do the children's sermons for March. He was so impressed he asked Sam to continue full time. God is so gracious! Sam says he will do the sermons as long as God feeds him the ideas. Many times he doesn't get the idea until he is sitting in church prior to the time to talk. And every one of his sermons are so insightful. I know he is in God's hands.

Well, it's six o'clock. I've been up since one–thirty. I went to bed at ten–thirty with a little back pain but nothing that would keep me from sleeping. At one o'clock, I woke up with my hips burning and the burn streaking down to my calves (both sides: on a pain scale of 1–10, I was a solid 8. I emailed Dr. Rosenfeld at two o'clock. He talked to me Friday at the clinic about my back pain. He discussed putting me on Tegretol or Dilantin since I am already on Neurontin. It's sounding like I have inflamation of my sciatic nerves. It still hurts to sit very long and reclining is impossible. Therefore, I'm not very helpful at the hospital, unless they want to pay me to give out hugs. (Run that by Barbara and see what she thinks. Ha ha ha)

My daughter, Sara, had an interview at Medical College of Ga Physical Therapy Dept. last week. To make it all the way to the interview is pretty good. She is hedging a bit due to the cost, but we will do whatever we have to in order to allow her to go to school. Please keep us and her in your prayers. I pray every day for God to guide my children and to keep them close and I see His hand at work.

Well, that's the news. Sam and Alan are bummed at going back to school today. I checked with Alan and this computer doesn't have the fax receiving program that our previous one had. Please ask Valerie to show you how to get into the email program in the computer in the station where she was working when in your office. That way we can better talk. You email me, I send a message right back to you. That's the way I communicate with the world. If not, I'll have my Lightwriter and speaker set up for calls so you can give me a call. Either way, I look forward to your message. Have a blessed Monday—I know they may be mutually exclusive.

Kugs and hisses, _____ *and* _____
DC

Will and Taylor are Catherine's nephews, so she and Larry came to our church for their baptism. Those two boys are definitely one–hundred–percent BOYS.

From: Alan & Debra Coleman Home Fax
To: Catherine Parnell
April 13, 1999

Oh Catherine!
I have a joke for you.

A woman died and found herself standing outside the Pearly Gates, being greeted by St. Peter. She asked him, "Oh. Is this place really what I think it is? It's so beautiful. Did I really make it to heaven?"

To which St. Peter replied, "Yes, my dear. These are the gates to heaven. But you must do one more thing before you can enter." The woman was very excited, and asked of St. Peter what she must do to pass through the gates.

"Spell a word," St. Peter replied.

"What word?" she asked.

"Any word," answered St. Peter, "It's your choice."

The woman promptly replied, "Then the word I will spell is love. L-O-V-E." St. Peter congratulated her on her good fortune to have made it to heaven, and asked her if she would mind taking his place at the gates for a few minutes while he took a break. "I'd be honored," she said, "But what should I do if someone comes while you are gone?" St. Peter reassured her and instructed the woman simply to have any newcomers to the Pearly Gates spell a word as she had done. So the woman is left sitting in St. Peter's chair and watching the beautiful angels soaring around her, when low and behold, a man approaches the gates and she realizes it is her husband.

"What happened?" she cried, "Why are you here?"

"I was so upset when I left your funeral I was in an accident. And now I am here. Did I really make it to heaven?"

To which the woman replied, "Not yet. You must spell a word first."

"What word?" he asked.

The woman responded, "Czechoslovakia."

Love and Laughter,
Debra C.

Date: Wed 14 Apr 1999 10:26

Oh Al!
I'm drunk as a skunk on that Tegretol. I took it at 8:00, then slept from
8:30 until 10:00 when I woke up to shouting voices on the Jenny Jones
show. Uuuuggghhhh!!!!!!!!!

I know with the Flexeril it put me out at first, then its sedative effects
lessened, but I can't walk down the hall without hitting the walls. You
would scream with laughter. I want to go outside and play in the dirt
but I'm scared to do that. Other than the sedation, it relaxes the muscles. So if I did fall, I wouldn't be able to get up. So stop laughing!! And
don't call me your drunk ole' bag at home.

Regarding the Flonase. I just need it through the high pollen because I
think the sinus drainage is partly the cause of some of my throat
spasms.

Well that's all I can type. I need to find a horizontal surface.

Wovingly, laggeringly, and stoozy,
_____ _____ *and* _____
Dink—I THINK

Dink was one of those people who almost never took any kind of medica-
tion beyond the occasional aspirin. Before she got sick, when she would
have sinus problems and need to take an antihistamine, she would only
take half of the normal adult dosage, yet it would wipe her out for two

days. Not surprisingly, some of the stronger meds she had to take with the disease gave her experiences like she had never dreamed of before.

Date: Thu 15 Apr 1999 09:46

Oh Alan,
I assume I drove you out with my sounds. I'm so sorry and it's about time. Just kidding.

Woke up at 8:30. I'm still woozy. Managed a shower and getting dressed. The grab bars, towel rack, and sink came in handy.

I'm really seeing weakness in my left quad today. Especially when I was getting dressed, can we absolutely write it down and do some work on it?

Got an email from Cindy Buckner. She just forgot and wants to set up another date. I told her I would talk with you and let her know.

I guess I slept through the rain. In my dream, I worked on plastic rings putting flowers on them. But there was some problems about how to put them on and in what designs. So I fussed all night. What did you do?

As opposed to a trache, I want to explore taking out my vocal cords, that way they couldn't close and we both could sleep happier.

Well, enough chatter. Hurry home. I need a giant hug.

Gugless and hoozy,   _____ *and* _____
D   N
   I   K

Cindy Buckner is a nurse with the Georgia ALS Association who provides in-home consulting and patient care for PALS (People with ALS). She is a wonderfully caring and knowledgeable person who could use a good assistant. With so much on her schedule, she accidently forgot an appointment with us. No harm done.

We had been advised that one way to eliminate the noises Dink made when she exhaled was to have a tracheotomy. That way, the air could pass in and out of her lungs without passing through her throat. Traches can be messy and require a good bit of effort to maintain, so she was thinking "Why don't we just take the vocal cords out and solve the problem that way?"

Date: Thu 15 Apr 1999 13:04

OK ITS 1:00 AND I'M STILL OUT OF IT.

YOU KNOW
H
    O
        O

Poor kid. Forgot the "W" and never even knew the difference.

Date: Fri 16 Apr 1999 09:52

Midmornin' babee,
I decided to reduce the dose of Tegretol to 200mg and see what that did. I also took Benadryl Allergy Sinus this morning with the lower dosed Tegretol. Well I just woke up from a hour and half nap. My legs are

stinging just a bit and my head is a whole lot better so I may take this 5 times a day today to see if it works.

It looks like a beautimous day outside. If possible I may try to get a few of those dangerous rays. I figure the odds of my getting melanoma are slim. Getting a boss tan compliments of Lou Gehrig. Thank you Lou! I know I'm being morbid. I'll stop.

Just think. In a few hours you can take that tie off, put some shorts on and just feel the freedom. Weekend's here!!!

Well hang in there, sweetie. I'll see ya soon.

Love,
Tan, svelt, and sexy at 110 Flint Hill Drive

Dink had always been very careful to avoid getting too much sun. She would almost always wear a hat when she was out in the yard and generally used tons of sun screen with SPF "Infinity" when she was at the beach. She would usually wear one-piece swim suits, although that had as much to do with her perception about her weight as it did with sun protection. I'm not real big on using cliches, but the old saying about making lemonade when life gives you lemons is just too appropriate to ignore here. The disease diminished the cancerous threat of the sun's rays for her and it caused her to lose some weight, so she went out and bought her first bikini in twenty years and proceeded to get a really nice tan. I gotta tell ya, she was lookin pretty hot that Spring. (And I'm sure my children just freaked out at hearing Dad say that about Mom. After all, parents don't think and talk about......THAT! Do they?)

Date: Fri 16 Apr 1999 11:08

Hey again,
I might as well tell you because you will see the blood on the carport. I
was coming back inside and I lost my balance so I grabbed at the
Camaro (which has nothing to grab onto) and I went down face first.
Assessment: I have just a small blue spot on the right bridge of my nose
but no displacement. And most of the blood came from both nostrils
bleeding. My upper lip is the size of Rhode Island. It is busted in three
or four places, but it's so swollen it's hard to tell. Teeth okay. Eyes okay.
Glasses just need an adjustment. Arms okay, hands okay. Legs okay.
Feelings bruised terribly.

I would say I'm sorry but I'm the one who fell. I'll see you when you get
home. I'm trying to ice my face.

Love,
BUWWA

*I didn't get this message before I got home that day so the first indication I
had that something was wrong was the pool of blood I found on the carport
floor. I rushed into the house and found her lying on the couch with most
of her face covered by an ice pack. She looked like she had been beaten. I
peppered her with questions to make sure there were no serious injuries
that would need medical attention and she convinced me there were none.
After I made sure she had everything she needed to be as comfortable as she
could be, I sat at the end of the couch with her legs in my lap and just
looked at her. She was OK, but all I could do was cry. I cried because she
was hurt and I cried because she was okay. I cried because I knew she
would fall again. I cried because I knew the measures we could take to keep
her from falling would also diminish her sense of independence. I cried
because I wasn't there. She knew better than to try to stop my crying before*

I got it all out, but when I had settled down somewhat she said, "Well, at least it's unanimous now." I didn't understand what she meant. "Now I've fallen in every room of the house INCLUDING the carport." I just shook my head…and stopped crying.

Of course, not all of her falls were so serious. She got up in the middle of one night to go to the bathroom and a few moments later I heard that unmistakable thud as she hit the floor. I jumped out of bed, dashed into the bathroom, threw the light switch on and looked around, fully expecting to find her with a broken neck or worse, but there was no Dink. Confused, I turned around and headed back into the bedroom and there she was…sitting IN THE UNPACKED SUITCASE that had been left on the floor at the foot of our bed. She waved at me to let me know she was OK, so I sat down in the suitcase with her and we both fell out, laughing our heads off.

From: Alan & Debra Coleman Home Fax
To: Catherine Parnell
April 18, 1999

Hey Caterina!
Dr. Rosenfeld put me on Tegretol 250 mg for my back and leg pain last Tuesday. It made me drunk as a skunk. I couldn't walk without hitting walls. So I emailed him Thursday and I started decreasing the dose myself. Friday morning I was doing much better. I went outside for just a minute. As I was walking back in I wobbled and reached out to steady myself on the rear of my son's very waxed sleek Camaro. Needless to say my hand slid right on down and I hit the carport cement. Impact point: face. To be more precise: my nose and mouth. No teeth broken but one huge fat upper lip and it looks more and more like my nose is broken. And you thought you had a busy week. I'm coming in Monday morning to get my snoz x-rayed. With any luck I can see Dr. Kaiser early Monday. Alan and I leave for Charlotte for my monthly injection. I have started a

lower dose of Tegretol with no appreciable problems but no help to back pain yet.

Sara is waiting to hear from Medical College of Ga. about acceptance. She has a spot at Ga State, but she really wants to go to Med. College.

So far, Joe is not on the list to go anywhere, but my cousin, Keith Wynn, or Skeeter, is headed to the desert so those guys can come home or go to Kosova.

We opened our big beautiful addition yesterday. It was awesome! I cried through the whole thing.

I'm hoping the medication will handle this "pain." I am pretty tired of it. I am also really tired of this house. I miss ya'll. I'll try to stop by to see you while there for the x-rays. Hang in there.

Snoken broz, _____ _____
Debra C.

Joe is in the Army Reserve and had been put on notice that he might have to ship out to any of a number of different overseas locations. We were quite anxious about that for a while, but thankfully he never had to go anywhere. Keith is a full time, career Marine and spent a while in the desert before coming back stateside to an assignment in Washington, DC.

Our church added a new building to house the fellowship hall, youth department and church offices. The church members did a lot of the cleanup and moving in, so we all had a sense of ownership in the new facility. We were especially proud of the fact we did this under an interim pastor and interim music minister. In fact, our youth minister was our only full time ministerial staff member. Ty Ragan, you did a marvelous job.

Date: Wed 21 Apr 1999 11:25

Hey Al,
Woke up a little after 4 and thought, "He must have been snoring very loud and didn't want to wake me." Ha-Ha. I would hear you snoring so I knew you were okay. I woke up around 5 and realized I was sleeping, not tossing. I didn't hear you come in, shower, dress, get your keys. I remember your kiss when I wanted to throw my arms around your neck but the body wasn't responding.

I have something I want you to print for me. It's an article on the Ride For Life web site. The topic is palliative care. I am so very interested in it.

Such a wonderful yesterday. The grass and steps were endearing.

MMMMMMMMMMMMMMMMMMMMMMMMMMMMMMMM
MMMMMMMMMMMMMMMMMMMMMMMMMMMMMMMM
MMMMMMMMMMMMMMMMMMMMMMMMMMMMMMMM
MMMMMMMMMMMMMMMMMMMMMMMMMMMMMMMM
MMMMMMMMMMMMMMMMMMMMMMMMMMMMMMMM
MMAHAHAHAHAHAHAHAHAHAHAHAHAHAHAHAHAHA
HAHHAHAHAHAHAHAHAHAHAHAHAHAHHAHAHAHHA
HAHHAHHAHAOOOOOOOOOOOOOOOOOOOOOOOOOOOO
OOOOOOOOOOOOOOOOOOOOOOOOOOOOOOOOOOOOO
OOOOOOOOOOOOOOOOOOOOOOOOOOOOOOOOOOOOO
OOOOOOOOOOOOOOOOOOOOWEEE

Thanks for driving.

Love overflowing, mushy, wistful, cozy love,
Dink

Lots of times, when I would be awakened repeatedly by her sighs, I would move into the den and spend the rest of the night on the coma-couch…but she could still hear my snoring from the other end of the house.

We had been in Charlotte the day before for a study visit. The appointment was routine and took less than an hour, so we should have been back home by supper time, but…

We had gone to Charlotte the night before the appointment and when I got back to the hotel after picking up supper, the radiator on the car blew out. Early the next morning, we called the ALS center and made arrangements for Ruth, the research assistant, to come get Dink. Then I rolled the dice and tried to limp the car to a garage where it could be repaired and, luckily, I made it.

The car wasn't ready until 5:00 that afternoon, so Dink and I spent the day hanging out with Sandy and the rest of Dr. Rosey's staff. It was a beautiful day so we spent a couple of hours sitting on the lawn outside. It was really neat because the grass was overdue for a mowing so it was long and soft and made for a childlike afternoon of reading, talking and spotting cloud shapes. There was also a set of stairs nearby, so we did some stair laps to work on her leg strength some. We couldn't have had a better day.

Date: Fri 23 Apr 1999 06:29

If you are going to stack the deck and take that nasal inhaler and sleep propped on two pillows, this is not a valid test. Go back to sleeping normally. I won't send you to Kaiser yet, but you have to agree to a daily routine in which you start and do lose weight. I will continue to sleep elsewhere.

I'm not going to go any further with this email.

Fold coes torever,
Dink

Oh my goodness. That was a spanking. Dink got the notion that maybe my own snoring was waking me as much as her loud sighs were. To find out, she would sleep in Sara's room and see whether it effected my rest. The problem was she didn't tell me it was a test. She just said, "I'm going to sleep in Sara's room to see if you can sleep better." I thought she meant I was SUPPOSED to sleep better, so I took a couple of other measures to insure I did. Oh, was I ever so wrong. The mandate to lose weight was aimed at reducing my soft-nasal-tissue-induced snoring that most over-weight people experience. Sleeping elsewhere was temporary, but I'm still trying to lose that weight.

Date: Mon 26 Apr 1999 06:58

Hey sweetie,
I was thinking this morning and you know how dangerous that is. I think you need to keep an eating diary for a week or two so we can look into areas we can improve. I know the sausage egg and cheese biscuit from McDonald's is comfort food but it probably contains your whole day's calories. If you want, I can get the exact calories and fat grams for you. I suspect we have two areas of needed improvement.

When you don't eat at home, either the sec-biscuit has such a strong pull or you don't have time, which is it? If you had time would you eat cereal? Or is the sec the thing? And it's about time to cut back on the coffee and get back on the bicycle. It will be good for you and might get Sam back on the bike, if his bike still fits.

Well enough bashing. When I woke up at four, I wasn't feeling very much pain, but as I started to move, there it was. I had entertained ideas

of snuggling up to that point. Hope this is over soon. Have a great
Monday. Wrap yourself in the shield of hugs and kisses. I'll see you later.

All carm and wuddly,   *All _____ and _____*
Dink

*We had started a diet a few months before her diagnosis and we had some
success with it, but dieting and ALS do not mix. ALS increases your metabolism significantly, causing excessive weight loss, so one of the first things
Dr. Rosenfeld told her was to "maximize the caloric intake of EVERY bite
you put in your mouth." I, of course, felt obligated to support her in that
effort and what better way is there to support someone than to join them?
So my weight went up as hers went down. She was also concerned because
I was no longer riding my bicycle and my family histories include all the
bad things that result from being sedentary and overweight. To make
things worse, I was teaching at a school located about forty–five minutes
away from home, so I usually left by 6:30 AM to beat the traffic and have
some quiet time to prepare for the day. I had discovered that eating a biscuit as I drove to work saved time and helped me stay awake for the drive.
I never objected to eating cereal, I just didn't want to get up early enough to
have time to eat at home and then end up starting the drive on a full stomach. It was one of those issues we never resolved.*

Date: Mon 26 Apr 1999 11:58

Here again,
Slept all the way through Regis and Kathy Lee. Yeaaaaaaaa! I also found
out I can eat a boiled egg chopped up when I can't eat a scrambled egg.
Weird! I have all the machines, except the vacuum, going. I worked you
over pretty strong earlier. But we both know since the weather is better,
it's time to git goin'.

I read my email from my cousin Margene Wynn. She's Aunt Myrl's daughter and our first cousin. It's her son who has been shipped to Kuwait. He's career Marine. Loves it. Go figure. She filled in a big chunk in my family's health history. We need to work on yours for Sam. And I need to write Myrtis and Clyde about their's. Sara had mentioned this a few months ago.

Well, gotta go. The darlins are on Andy Griffith. Guitar playing galore! Yeah!

Love and snikles, (couldn't exchange that)
Dink

Myrtis and Clyde Hobby are Alan Hobby's parents. If I had to choose a second set of in-laws, I couldn't do any better than them. Despite the fact I was wearing blown out blue jeans and a sweaty old t-shirt the very first time we met, I have always felt completely accepted and loved by them. In fact, when we would visit them in South Florida, they would introduce us as their daughter and son-in-law. That was always important, and it deeply touched Dink. The kids put a novel twist on their situation. By the time Dink came into my life, my parents had divorced and both had remarried, so counting them, Dink's parents and the Hobbys, the kids thought they were really lucky because they had eight grandparents. I couldn't agree more.

Date: Mon 26 Apr 1999 13:15

Me again,

Dr. Rosenfeld emailed me back. He thought I was already on Dilantin. He also mentioned some ALSers had their vocal cords sutured, which was less invasive. But he said he would investigate the cord removal. He asked about my vocalizations and I filled him in to every nook and cranny. I will let you know if I need you to pick up another prescription.

Hope your day is going great. I'm sorry you had to work at home so long. And I'm sorry I wasn't much help. But I want to share my notes from church. Len was very interesting. His sermon was on when not to pray. Wow! At least I didn't cry through the whole thing.

We need to think about changing the sign in the next day or two. The day is dreary but nice and cool with a nice breeze. Get out for a few minutes if you are going to have a long day. Feel it.

Blankity-blank.
Suppressed,
Dink

Date: Mon 26 Apr 1999 13:23

OH YEAH. YOU ATE ALL THE LIMA BEANS. I HAVE NONE TO EAT.

LOVE,
GROWLING STOMACH

Oops! Busted.

Date: Tue 27 Apr 1999 07:48

Mornin' sweetheart,
Maybe that's the temporary answer. As long as I am getting up at four, I can just make contact with you around five. Sound ok? I took some Tegretol at four so I'm a little bleary eyed right now.

I know you'll find my numerous emails from yesterday, today. I just talked my head off.

I saw the greatest news on the TV this morning. I knew there was some use of fetal cells being implanted in the brains of Parkinson's Disease patients with remarkable results. There is talk of trying it with ALS. Ooooooooooooowwwwwwwweeeee!! I do hope the research doesn't take 5 years.

Anyway. When Cindy Buckner finally gets here and we discuss some stuff, I want you to talk to the kids about how they feel about my end of life possibilities and maybe you talk with Len or someone and then let's me and you have an absolutely honest one–on–one and hammer this thing out. I want you to be absolutely honest because I know your future is very bright.

Well, to fluffier stuff. Where are we going to put all this stuff? I am going to have to revise some of the kitchen I guess. Gotta hit the bathroom. Bye!!

Love and tight spoonin,
Dink

If you could ask her to name one thing she had wanted to do, but never did, she would likely say, "Have that 'end of life possibilities' talk we never got around to." If you were to ask me to name one thing we did not do, that I am glad we did not do, I would say, "Have that 'end of life possibilities' talk we never got around to." She had made known to me and some of her friends at NGH, that she did not want any extreme measures taken to prolong her life artificially and I agreed wholeheartedly. I never pursued "hammering this thing out" though, because I knew if we did, it would lead to a discussion about funeral plans. In previous discussions from previous years, she had expressed a desire to be cremated, primarily to save the family the expense of traditional funeral arrangements. That seemed logical to me at that time, so if she had died unexpectedly in an accident of some sort, I probably would have honored that request. But things had changed.

Our fight against the disease was not a private fight. It had become a very public fight being waged by a massive army of people who loved her dearly. I knew in the end it would take a very public celebration of her life to help all of us begin to heal, so I did something I had tried to forget how to do: I totally avoided the issue with her. She may possibly have changed her mind by this time or been willing to say, "It's your decision," but I just could not chance that she would take a firm stand the other way.

Date: Tue 27 Apr 1999 15:35

HEY BABEE,
What's your ETA today?

LOVE,
Anxiously Waiting

Date: Tue 27 Apr 1999 15:42

OH,
Let me rephrase that. What's your ETA today?

LOVE,
Brost Aweathlessly Maiting   _____ _____ _____

From: Alan & Debra Coleman Home Fax
To: Catherine Parnell
April 29, 1999

Hey Catherine,
Where did this weather come from? Shouldn't it have been here in March when we were having 90's? We've got the heater running but Alan forgot to close the big two windows in the family room that were open the other wonderful day. Now they're swollen from the overnight rain we had so I can't get them closed. So I have fresh air on top of heated air. Healthy?

We saw Larry the other night when we stopped to pick up a refill. After the Tegretol wasn't working, Dr. Rosenfeld is putting me on Dilantin. How long have I been playing this game of convincing the Drs. of what it is and getting it successfully treated? Forever!! Haven't slept all the way through the night in months. Now I also have burning pain in my shoulders and elbows at a lower level during the day and raging at night. I'm just a mess! Did I tell you I was stooping to pick up something the other day and I tipped over front-ways and bopped my previously broken nose? Oh, a pair of Alan's shoes cushioned the fall but I bled for awhile. I told Alan to look at the bright side. At least I was zeroing in on my area for most possible fractures. Ha.

Well, that's about all from the Coleman ranch. Hope all is okay at NGH and with you. Give my love to all and I hope the Dilantin works. I miss ya'll.

Love and Hugs,
Debra C.

MAY 1999

Those Measly Squirrels

From: Alan & Debra Coleman Home Fax
To: Catherine Parnell
May 10, 1999

Hey Catherine,
It's another day in achesville. Had a wonderful weekend! Had all 3 kids here. With all the pollen, I have trouble with sinus drainage. I cough and wheeze, but Joe hadn't seen me do this, so he left the dinner table. Alan went with him and talked to him and he came back to the table and I talked to him. I assured him the sounds of "death" were only sinus trouble. Ha ha ha!!

I wish you had heard Sam's Mother's Day children's sermon. He said a mother's love is the closest thing to Jesus' love we have here on earth. He also said moms were equipped with a few other miracles. One being, the world's most powerful cleaner: Mom Spit. We rolled!!

Well I slept until 2 am when my "pun" started stinging. I toughed it out until 2:30 when my hips started stinging. I got up, took medicine, doodled around until 4:30, then back to bed, legs stinging, too. Tossed until around 6:00 then finally slept.

The only car here is the '71 Torino. Alan and Sam have forbidden me from driving it. I'm afraid I have to agree. Just getting it in gear is an ordeal.

Anyway, I'm going to get an appointment with Dr. Stillerman. He's had a couple of ideas that sound most appealing. Pain relief without being knocked out for 2 hours with every pill. That's been one of the hardest parts about working. Timing the pills so I don't fall prostrate on the floor and send Linda Lott into the heebee-geebees.

Well, that's enough. Hugs all around. Pray for me on all fronts. Oh! Joe turns 22 tomorrow. He gave up on school in the second grade so we fought an uphill climb. He was also in the gifted program but his artistic being never gelled with public school. Well, after two disastrous tries at college, he is back in school, Truett-McConnell. Straight A's!!! God does answer prayer!!

Gonna go. Pain in punsville.

Kove la yid,   _____ _____ _____
Debra C.
aka Dink

Date: Mon 10 May 1999 09:47
Subject: CRAZY TIMES

Hey darlin',
Weird night. Awake at 2:00 with back stinging. Up at 2:30 and took medication, answered email, faxed Dr. Stillerman, worked on the kitchen. Thought I was in the clear at 4:00 and came back to bed. But then my back, hips, and legs were stinging. The reverse snuggle was the

most comfortable position I could find. Still I only napped until after you left. When I came back to bed at 4:00, I was still planning to go to work but when it all unfolded I knew I couldn't. I just faxed Dr. Still.'s office staff for an appt. I asked for it to be after 2:30 any day.

I woke up around 8:30 and faxed Catherine. Opted for no shower just now. I'll clean up later. Still cloudy from the 2:30 medication. Dr. Stillerman's ideas would give me relief without this sleepiness!! Where do I sign up????

Our cat friend is walking across the yard. The yard is becoming truly beautiful. Birds all around, feasting on all those grass seeds you knocked down with the mower. You are my bird feeding competition!! No harm meant.

Hope your Monday is truly awe—inspiring. I swan! You have so many new projects on your agenda! I keep you in my prayers fervently!! I love you, my snuggle buddy.

Mistening to lusic and batching the wirds,
_____ to _____ and _____ the _____
Dink

We put three bird feeders out in the yard and had been experimenting with different types of food…sort of like you do with kids…trying to find out what they liked best. Maybe we should have raked up some of the grass clippings and put them in the feeders.

Date: Mon 10 May 1999 10:30
Subject: THOSE MEAZLY SQUIRRELS

Hey again,
I hate to tell you this, but the forward bird feeder is too close to the tree
trunk. The squirrel just jumps on top of the feeder. A good 1/4th of the
food has been consumed as of 10:00. We can work on this later today.
Fun, fun!

LOVE YA',
Dink

*OK. So we ended up having to put up one feeder dedicated exclusively to
the squirrels. It had a shelf at the bottom of its plexiglass front where the
squirrels could sit and see the food inside. The top was hinged and over-
hung the front, so the furry little fellas had to push the top up with their
nose to get to the peanuts inside. I never realized how diverse the squirrel
population is. We had a couple that acted as if they invented the whole
hinged-lid-feeder concept, snatching and eating peanuts at will. We also
had a couple that would have starved to death if our feeder had been their
only source of food, because the poor guys just could not figure out how it
worked. We didn't worry about them too much though, because we knew
they could always just jump on top of the bird feeder that was too close to
the tree.*

Date: Mon 10 May 1999 11:15

Hey one more time,
Dr. Stillerman wants me to see the pain clinic at NGH before I see him.
I am to call Michele at the pain clinic, at 770xyz0405. Set the appt. for
when it's convenient for you. Any info she wants that you don't know,
get her fax number and I'll fax it to her.

Wayne with Century 21 called. You can reach him this evening at 770xyz1169. Go tiger!!!

Hove mor fy lunk,   _____ _____ _____ _____
Dink

We had toyed for quite some time with the idea of getting an older house to fix up and rent out. I found one that looked interesting and had left a message with the realtor to call me back, but it turned out to be nicer than what we had in mind, though not as nice as what the sellers had in mind. That particular house would have been out of our budget though, even if they had not been asking too much for it. Actually, only a house in total shambles would have been in our budget, but it was still fun to talk about.

I think it was really important that we kept dreaming of the future like that. We knew the eventual outcome of the disease and had accepted it, but we also knew we had to keep on living in the meantime. If we had quit dreaming of the future, even though hers was limited, we would have been giving in to the disease, and we just refused to do that.

Date: Mon 10 May 1999 11:23

(Laughing),
Baby, let me know how much the percentage is of my emails in comparison to all your others.
Dink

The only reason it was not 100% was the two or three online subscriptions I had for news and investment services. None of those were ever as much fun to read though.

Date: Thu 13 May 1999 04:35
Subject: Re: Party with The Bigs

I wouldn't have had it any other way. They have had as much fun with
you as you have had with them. You're a very wonderful father. Just pray
for God's guidance and protection and be there for the highs and lows
and anything in between.

I LOVE YOU 2,
Dink

*When the kids were younger, we gave Joe and Sara the collective nickname
"The Bigs." As in, "You stay with the baby and I'll take The Bigs to a
movie."*

*Joe's birthday is May 11, so I had taken him and Sara and her boyfriend
out to eat. Sam couldn't go because he had to work and Dink wouldn't go
because she didn't want to take away any of the attention Joe should be getting on his big day. She was very aware that any time she and I were
together, I was totally pre-occupied with tending to her but she wanted me
to be able to give that attention to Joe instead. We finished eating and got
home early enough to spend some time with her, so I didn't feel too bad
about leaving her at home. Anyway, I emailed her on May 12, bemoaning
the fact she hadn't been with us, but telling her how much fun we had at
the restaurant and how thankful I was she had brought Joe and Sara into
my life.*

JUNE 1999

She Became My Caregiver

Date: Wed 02 Jun 1999 07:13

Mornin sweetie,
Hope the day is wonderful. If you come home early, and you don't mind my coming home too, call me. Of course if a nap is what you want, don't call.

Sorry I bugged out on you last night but I couldn't find the skeeter spray.

See you later,
I love yous—Dink

I never "minded" her coming home, but she knew that the best way for me to get a restful nap was to be at home alone.

One of the toughest things to do as a caregiver is to balance your own physical and emotional needs with those of the person you're caring for. It's especially hard if that person is a close loved one. I always felt guilty when I would do anything that was not directly related to her care and I often felt like I shouldn't do something fun that she could no longer do. I know now, it was vitally important to do those things anyway, and it seems so blatantly obvious that if I didn't take care of myself, I wouldn't have been able to take care of her. But it's nearly impossible to see that when you're caught up in the throes of the day-to-day details of caring for someone you love so much who has such a catastrophic disease. What is amazing to me still, is that she knew that, and so knowing, became MY caregiver. I don't think anybody else could have helped me survive Dink's disease better than Dink did.

From: Alan & Debra Coleman Home Fax
To: Catherine Parnell
June 24, 1999

Hey Cat-sister,
Feelin' kinda stove up post tumble. Hangin' at thuh hood 4 2-day, got it, chick? Nothing serious, so don't go over the deep end, okay Mom? Anyway, tell Quinn the cancer packet is ready except for copying cover letter and log. Anyway, it will be ready to go out Monday after her review. Thanks, seestah.

Firmly in His Hands,
Debra—The Weeble—Coleman

SUMMER 1999

Mama! There's a Man!

Since school was out, there were no emails during the summer of 1999. It was actually a very good summer. We took a trip down to Naples to visit with Myrtis and Clyde and had a laugh along the way. Somewhere along the vast stretches of I-75 in southwestern Florida, Dink told me she needed to visit the little girls room. We stopped at a Wendy's in a small town whose name I can't remember and went inside to take care of business. She had reached the point she needed help with her clothes, as well as getting on and off the toilet, so our first decision was which public restroom would be graced with the presence of the opposite of its intended gender. She insisted on the "Ladies" room because she thought it would be cleaner than the "Mens." I think there was a sexist attitude in there somewhere, but you can't really argue with the truth. We stopped a lady who was coming out of the restroom and asked her to do a little reconnaissance for us to make sure we didn't surprise any unsuspecting patrons who might still be inside. She assured us the coast was clear. We made our way into one of the stalls and as we were accomplishing the task at hand, we heard a couple of ladies come in, do their thing, then leave again, never knowing there was anything out of the ordinary going on. As we were about to exit the stall we heard another lady come in, so I whispered, "Let's let her get finished and out the door." So we waited a couple of minutes, trying not to get tickled, until finally we had our chance to escape. About that time though, we heard a lady come in to the restroom with at least two, but possibly three, kids in tow. We just looked at each other, smiled a little, and shrugged our shoulders, then I said, "Well, we can't stay in here forever." So we bopped out of the stall before any of our new potty pals could start dropping their drawers.

The expression on the face of the first little girl that saw us was priceless. She appeared startled, but not afraid, as she exclaimed, "Mama, there's a man!"

Of course, the mother quickly spun around to see what her daughter was talking about and, seeing Dink, said, "It's okay, honey, hold the door open for them." The little girl obliged, but she kept her eyes intently on me, occasionally glancing back at her mother to make sure it was still okay. I thanked the mother and the daughter as the door was closing behind us and just as it was about to shut completely, I gave the little girl a big, exaggerated wink.

As we were pulling away in the car, I told Dink, "I wonder how many more times we'll get to do that." She just laughed.

The stay in Naples was very restful and relaxing. As far as I can remember, it was the only time we went down there without the kids. That gave us a chance to really visit with Myrtis and Clyde, so we spent a lot of time talking with them and playing cards and hanging out by the pool. The pool was great. Dink could stand up and walk in the water with me only holding her hand. We tried, once, for me to let go, but she started sinking quickly, so we knew we had to maintain contact. With that in mind, we just spent a lot of time holding hands, walking around in the pool, flirtin and courtin and being close, just like we'd done a thousand times in the past.

We also extended one of our Charlotte trips. I can't remember if it was a clinic visit or a study visit, but we left home a couple of days early and traveled up the east coast of South Carolina, then stayed at Myrtle Beach in a hotel overlooking the ocean. The next day we took a large ferry boat ride near Cape Fear, North Carolina, then headed toward Charlotte from Wilmington. It was another great time for us as we traveled at our own pace and stopped to check out anything that looked interesting. It was one of the "good" experiences we had that most likely would not have happened, had it not been for the disease.

By the time school started again in August, Dink could no longer drive. In fact, her last time at the wheel was quite an adventure. In July, Sam and I took his car to a garage in Conyers on the day before he left for a week-long mission trip with the church youth group. Now, Conyers is about fifteen miles from our house, and most of that is interstate, so it's not such a bad drive, but Dink's left arm was weak and she had already begun having problems turning her head to the right. Of course, the shop called after a couple of days to tell us the car was ready, and Dink insisted she could drive it back if I would take her out there to get it. One of my biggest problems during the disease was my inability to tell her "No." Especially, "No. You can't do that anymore." So off we went to Conyers.

After we got her situated in Sam's car, I walked all the way around it, trying to determine if she could see me the whole time. We discovered she did have one "blind spot," namely oncoming traffic to her immediate right, but she insisted on driving anyway so we improvised our way home. Driving my car, I lead her out of the garage parking lot and became "Officer Al" by pulling into and stopping slightly to the right of each intersection we came to, blocking any traffic from that side. She motored on through the intersection with only a slight decrease in speed, then I would catch up to her, pass her, and set up for her at the next intersection…all the way home, at every intersection. By the time we got home, we were both totally stressed out. Before getting out of the car she said, "Don't worry. We won't do that anymore."

My reply was "Thank you," but my relief was overshadowed by knowing the full implication of what she had just said. She never drove again.

Since she could no longer drive, we had to make arrangements to get her to work each morning when school started. I changed schools for the 1999–2000 school year which was good and bad. The good part was my new school being located only twenty minutes from home as opposed to the forty–five minute drive to my previous school. The bad part was the morning start time of my new school. Because class started at 7:20, I had to be signed in by 7:00, which put me on the road by 6:30, which was too early to drop her off at the hospital. Fortunately, we were saved by our neighbor, Vicky Rider. Vicky lives in our neighborhood, works at NGH in the business department, and agreed to become Dink's chauffeur. She would get her to work in the mornings and I would pick her up in the afternoons. This arrangement provided Vicky with a pretty nice perk: she got to park in Dink's prime location, Employee of the Year, reserved parking spot. If there could be such a thing as an Assistant Employee of the Year, Vicky would get my vote forever.

Another adjustment we had to make in the new school year was the increasing amount of time it took Dink to get ready for work. Even though she was getting up earlier, she just didn't have enough time to sit down and write an "AM EM" to me, so she changed her audience. The office where she did most of her work had no Internet connection, but it was on the NGH intra-net, so she began emailing her buddies there at the hospital. At the time, I really hated it, because I wasn't getting those regular "pick-me-ups" from her, but in retrospect, I'm glad I could share her thoughts and wit with those people at NGH who shared so much of themselves with us. As it turned out, Catherine Parnell saved most of the messages she got from Dink and was gracious enough to share them with me. What follows is the compilation of those messages.

AUGUST 1999

Floppy Mae Looks Irritated

From: DColeman
To: CParnell
Date: 8/20/99 9:49am

Mornin' glowree!
How's yer teeth hangin' on dis Fridee? Mine ain't so good. I got news my
Mama was gonna hafta hav a root kennel. I'm besides mysef. Why my
Mama? She's sucha good wooman ta hafta go throo dis. I have menny
kweschuns an the most impowtent one is what does dogs hafta do with
root kennels? If yous knows pleez send me infermashun.

Yors trooly,
Floppy Mae

*I really don't know what happened here or what brought this on, but Dink
developed an alter ego. I'm not sure, but my best guess is it happened like
this: Like a lot of people facing catastrophic, permanent challenges, Dink
turned to humor to help her cope with things. You've seen that in a number
of the messages you have already read. She also used it to put people at ease
when they were around her. Since her ALS progression began with bulbar
palsy, she lost the muscularity in her lips very early in the disease and they
drooped very noticeably. By August of 1999, her left arm was completely*

weakened and her feet had weakened to the point she had to wear braces for her ankles. In her comedic frame of mind, she was "floppy," and in a literal sense, she was indeed. So, "floppy" needed a proper name, and what else could you choose besides "Floppy Mae?" Of course, Floppy Mae would need a persona, and there could be none better than an Old South/Gullah/Creole/Appalachian/Carribean Islander mix. Right? Thus, Floppy Mae was born. Hey, it makes perfect sense to me.

From: DColeman
To: CParnell
Date: 8/25/99 8:58am

Dis iz to all ya'll deezasster folks Hicki Slider, Katreena Perrnall, 'n Beberlee Hol-lotta-shakin,

Whut kinna deezaster is ya'lles habin'. I had me wun jes de odder day. Me 'n my mayn skweeze, Al-eegater, wuz gittin rady fer werk. Now I'ded jes got me a new brazeer. I took its outta thuh box 'n started tryin' ta put hit on. Oh my buzzerd! I ain't never seesa such. Hit diden looky lik no brazeer. Al-eegater tried his bestes but hees jes a man-folk. Dem guyz dont know nuttin 'bout no brazeers cept taykin'em off. 'N sum nownsents 'bout how fastes day kin doo dat.

Well I struggld wit hit 'n finlee desided I needed ta read de dictshuns. Ever herd' o dis? Front closure wunder bra?

Yors tooly,
Floppy Mae

FYI: Hicki Slider is Vicky Rider…Katreena is Catherine Parnell…Beberlee is Beverly Holcomb, one of Dink's buddies from Medical Records. All are

part of the Disaster Response Team and probably had been paged over the
hospital's public address system.

From: DColeman
To: CParnell
Date: 8/27/99 9:04am

Jes hows yous ladees taday,
Hits Fridee. Halla looya! I herrs Valrees gonna leter har down 'n dust wit
dem kerls 'n I node Katreen kips her har short so's shes kin spike hit on
da weekens. I node her'n her feller, Hairy Pernail 'r gonna go ta da
soomo pig wreslin kontess dis weeken. oo-wee! Fun a' poppin! 'N I
heered Valree 'n Slik wuz goin ta werk on thems tans down at thuh
newkleer plant. Dem jet setters! As fer me 'n mine wees goona wach
thuh paint peel.

Well hopes yor weeken his funner dan a sloo 'o' monkees.

Sinseerlee,
Floppy Mae

From: DColeman
To: CParnell
Date: 8/27/99 10:04am

This is Debra, not Floppy. I sent her to catch flies in the O.R. And told
her not to come back until she caught five.

Here's the Debra mobility story. Just before we left on our trip South at
the end of July, I started a new medication that made me a little more
wobbly. This is common at the start of this kind of medication but it
usually subsides. Well, Alan is very afraid I'll fall and break my right

arm, which would be a disaster, I know. On the trip, he didn't let me walk alone ever. He would stand behind me and grab me around the waist and hold my right arm every time I walked. And most chairs are too low for me to get up unassisted. So Alan had total control over my comings and goings. When we got back, he surprised me with this wheelchair. Mind you we had tried canes and walkers, none helped. The canes were cumbersome and kept me leaning over. And I can't lift a walker with my left hand/arm and a walker wouldn't help when I did my "fall back" thing. So I accepted the wheelchair. Actually I felt imprisoned and went through an emotional upheaval.

This past Monday, in Charlotte, we reported the wobbliness. Dr. Rosenfeld listened about that, why I had the wheelchair, and about Alan's fears. He said, "But you still have good leg muscles and I want you using them. Hang on. I want you to try something." He left and brought back a similar walker to the one I have now. I got up and tried it and walked stabley down the hall to the PT room. There he had me try three other kinds of rolling walkers. The difference with these are brakes which I need on inclines to maintain control. And they can lock down for even better stability. Alan was impressed with my walk using these and got all excited. The model I have is the "New, improved '99 model." I accused Dr. Rosey of being a used car salesman in disguise. Of course, after weeks in that chair my muscles need to recover but I'm less worn out each day. I truly missed walking. There's so much independence in that one feat. (No pun intended) No, break it down more. Independent mobility. Because even an electric wheelchair serves that purpose.

Well there's the story. Uh-oh! Here comes Floppy looking irritated. Bye

DC

*One of the hardest things about being the primary caregiver for someone
you love is accepting the fact you can't be everything or do everything they
need. I was constantly battling with the inner turmoil of balancing her
need to feel independent with her need to be kept safe. She was absolutely
right, if she had fallen and broken her right arm, it would have been disastrous. What little independence she had, including her ability to communicate, was based entirely on her capacity to use her right arm. She was
naturally right-handed, so I knew if she fell, she would instinctively put
that hand out to stop the fall. Any time, no, EVERY time she was standing,
even with the walker, I was a nervous wreck. I still wish I could have
resolved that issue, but I never did.*

*If I could rescript our entire experience, one change I would make is
alluded to in this message. I would have gotten her a power wheelchair
very early. We were encouraged to wait, so she would be forced to use her
leg muscles and keep them viable longer. I think we would have been better
advised to go ahead and get a power chair (you have to be careful not to
call them electric chairs) so she could zip around anywhere she wanted.
Then she would have been less tired from "moving around" and we could
have pursued a physical therapy regimen to work on her leg muscles. In
fact, with a van that could transport her in the chair, anybody could have
taken her to the hospital for physical therapy, so we would not have been
limited by my schedule and availability. Just a little hind-sight.*

I'm in a Win-Win Situation

From: DColeman
To: CParnell
Date: 9/1/99 12:28pm

Hey Zipper Innocent,
Vicki Rider told me Barbara was concerned about my getting fatigued
here at work and that adversely affecting my immune system. On the
contrary, being here boosts my immune system because I love it here. I
go on the energy I glean from those around me, so I seldom get tired. If
I poop out, I sit back and breathe deep. If I'm really feeling bad I have an
army of Moms that can skirt me away. But even tired I feel better here
than home alone. If I am tired of work, I clock out and piddle around til
time to leave.

So there you are. My secret for livin' on love.

Debra C.

*Dink and Catherine developed a number of nicknames for each
other...you'd just have to know the two of them to understand why. I think
"Zipper Innocent" had to do with Catherine's having to do battle with one
of Dink's zippers when she was helping her in the bathroom.*

Barbara Valentine is the Nursing Services Administrator at the hospital. The rest of the message speaks for itself very nicely.

From: DColeman
To: CParnell
Date: 9/7/99 11:20am

Hey sis,
Serious note here. (Floppy Mae hasn't recovered from extra lazy days over the weekend.) Is it possible for me to get a password of my own to access the Internet so I can talk to Alan during the day? I think it could be approved because while others can talk with their families on the phone, I can't. Tell whoever I promise not to surf any. Thanks.

Firmly in His Hands,
Debra C.

If she had gotten Internet access, and could have written me every day, we probably wouldn't have the rest of these emails to enjoy. I've found these messages to be just as helpful to my healing as the ones she sent to me, because these show a side of her that probably would not have been expressed to me. To whomever made the decision not to give her a password: if you've been feeling guilty about that…let it go.

From: DColeman
To: CParnell
Date: 9/8/99 3:11pm

Hey Katreen,
This is Floppy. I herd 'bout da oppice shuffle perposall 'n thought dat da offending party shud vacate an let dem por coders we put in da closet hab a nice oppice wit air 'n all. Doncha tink?

Floppy Mae

This is my girl at her very best. There were a couple of people she had worked with, doing chart coding, that were literally working in a converted closet. Of course, closets don't have air conditioning registers or returns, so they get very stuffy. Dink was lobbying for her closet-mates to be moved into an office that was rumored to be coming available, although she no longer worked in the closet with them and would have gotten no benefit from the move. With all that was going on in her life, she was always watching out for ways to help other people.

From: DColeman
To: CParnell, JDieringer, KGillespie, VKordys, VPatrick...
Date: 9/9/99 10:20am
Subject: Debra Coleman's yuk yuk

Hey,
I thought of a cute joke I heard and I hope I don't slaughter it.

A grandfather had his granddaughter sitting on his lap. They were just 'a talking. The little girl studied his face and asked, "Why is your face so wrinkley?"

He answered, "Well, God made me a long time ago. That's why I have wrinkles. God made you, too. But you are newer."

The little girl solemnly considered his answer and said, "Well, He must have improved a lot since he made you."

Okay, okay. No boos or hisses.

I love ya'll,
Debra C.

From: DColeman
To: CParnell
Date: 9/9/99 l0:36am

Bessie belle!
I jes fownd yer email 'bout my harey laigs 'n Lex's katerax. So soree I misst it. As fer my laigs, I hav decided ta stop shavin' dem. My husbeen has ta shav dem 'n my under arms. Ta do dis I hafta strex out on da bed 'n he flips me around. What do ya tink 'bout my permenent hariness?

Luvinlee,
Floppy Mae

We rationalized on several occasions that her permanent hairiness was acceptable since certain European women don't shave under their arms, but are still considered sexy. With all due respect to sexy European women, I'm glad I live in the US.

From: DColeman
To: CParnell
Date: 9/10/99 12:23pm

I remembered it. Michele Bryant in business office sent it to me.

In Alabama, what is the difference in a divorce and a tornado? Nothing. You lose yer trailer in both.

Hold the applause, pleez.

DC

Apparently, she had told Catherine she heard a good joke but couldn't remember it. When she told me the same joke, I asked her if she knew the Alabama State Motto: "At least we ain't Mississippi!" If you don't follow Southeastern Conference college football, or if you're from Alabama or Mississippi, you may not appreciate the humor here. Trust me, though, it's very funny.

Go Dawgs…sic'em…woof, woof, woof!!!

From: DColeman
To: CParnell
Date: 9/13/99 5:17pm

Hit's me again,
I now also need to communicate with the head office of the cancer registry. They have email and I'd like to get an account on Judy's computer. Who do I talk to about this?

DC—ppps

She was persistent with her Internet password request and they were just as persistent in not giving her one.

"ppps" had nothing to do with the traditional Post Script you find at the end of some letters. Actually, she and Catherine had worked out a code so she didn't have to come right out and say "I need a potty break." They even devised a way for her to communicate the nature of the potty break she needed as well as the urgency of each request. I told her I thought that was pretty darn clever.

From: DColeman
To: KGillespie, QMcCoy, CParnell
Date: 9/14/99 4:12pm

This is to inform you that September 21, 1999, you will not have the pleasure of my obnoxious company. That delight will be conferred on the Carolinas ALS clinic where I will get my pump refilled with obnoxious fluid. That's where I get my pep so I can pester ya'll. In my absence, the Covington Police Department has agreed to pick up a few drunkerds (in the dear Dr.'s words) for Nursing II. The Alzheimer support group members have agreed to have their Alzheimer afflicted family members call the physician referral line. And I won't have to bother with Quinn. She is already covered in obnoxiousness with the Medscribe Program and the dictating program and the $ guys and I'll be here the 20th and I'll be back on the 22nd.

Firmly in His Hands,
Debra Coleman

From: DColeman
To: CParnell
Date: 9/17/99 8:48am
Subject: hairy

Catherine!
It's Fry-dee'!!! Just thought you might need reminding, I mean considering your gray hair and the fact you live with Larry Parnell. No, I'm not saying you're old. I may have thought it but I'm not voicing it. Nah, yer a sprang chikin'. The biggest reason I'm writing is that I'm wearing my flirty skirt today and I wanted you to see my hairy laigs. Way cool!! I'll see you later my ppp sister, but only pp today, thank you Father!

Firmly in His Hands,
DC

From: DColeman
To: CParnell
Date: 9/20/99 12:47pm
Subject: gray Monday yuk yuk

Two old ladies, Catherine and Barbara, were on a driving trip.
Catherine was driving and suddenly Barbara noticed she had run a red
light. Giving her friend the benefit of the doubt, Barbara thought she
had looked up too late to see it correctly. They kept driving. Suddenly,
Barbara looked up as they drove under the second red light. She was
alarmed but thought maybe it was a late yellow light Catherine ran, so
Barbara determined to pay close attention to Catherine's driving. At
this, Catherine ran the third red light.

"Catherine! What are you doing? You just ran three red lights!" Barbara
exclaimed.

Catherine replied, "Oh. Was I driving?"

Mirth per DC

From: DColeman
To: CParnell
Date: 9/22/99 9:16am
Subject: stuff

Mornin' glow-ree!!
Wednesday—yuk. Bosses gone—whoopeeee!!! As per our last discussion—1 sided—Monday. Re: bras and boob sizes, 36 DD…Al's a happy

boy. Visit to Charlotte went fine. This was just the injection day. I go to the all day clinic with all the specialists every 3 months. I go next, October 22. Oh, Catherine, I will be gone October 22 for clinic. I was weighed. 139–1/4. I have gained 2 lbs a week since changing my formula to a higher calorie brand. Now my pants are tight, cheeks pumped, breasts rounder and stand-upper, belly flopping. The latter has caused me to go on a diet. I want to hang in at 130–135lbs. So I've gone from 2700 cal/day to 1900 cal/day. I hope to go down a little then I'll go up till I stabilize.

I talked to the Dr. about the sudden change in my walking: slower, sloppier. I think it's the medicine I take for night time leg jumping. He said it could also be that the med took the stiffness out of my legs so I had to rely only on the muscles to pick up the extra load. Problem is, I wasn't stiff. I've seen stiff legs and mine were flexible. We'll continue our discussion via email, for example, last Friday no trouble getting into Vicki's van. Sunday I stumbled around all day. Monday I couldn't stand up after my foot was on the step of the van. Poor Vicki sweated. Same today. ALS isn't that fast. Well enough. See ya later.

Firmly in His Hands, (where he picks me up when I stumble)
DC

Ladies and gentlemen, if you think your spouses don't tell their friends your personal secrets, you might want to reread those first two lines. And I thought only guys talked that way.

We finally stabilized her weight around 130 pounds with a daily intake of 2400 calories. Keep in mind, she was getting no physical activity beyond walking to and from the car. As you can see, ALS does strange things to one's metabolism. By this point in time, Dink was using the PEG for all of her intake. Her nutritional supplement came in 8–ounce cans, each one containing 400 calories, and was available by prescription only. (Actually, in her case, it was erroneous to call it a supplement, because it was the only nutrition she was getting.) It was in the form of a "delicious chocolate shake" which was very thick, but not very delicious, so I was glad she had the feeding tube so she didn't have to endure the stuff by mouth. The supplement was so thick we had to dilute it almost 30% with water in order to get it to flow through the PEG, so she ended up getting 24 ounces of fluid at each meal, plus the water in which her meds were dissolved. She often told me she felt like her eyeballs were floating.

From: DColeman
To: CParnell
Date: 9/22/99 9:32am
Subject: stuff -reply -reply
Re: Stumbles.

My pastor has gone on and on about my being careful not to fall. I finally told him to hush! If I fall, I just fall. Not the end of the world. If I fall and I'm injured fatally, then I win. Glory sooner. You see, I am in a win-win situation. Now YOU hush!

Firmly in His Hands,
DC

This is the summation of her entire attitude regarding our experience with ALS. It was the basis of the strength we both needed in order to survive the disease. If I had to identify a single defining statement for our story, this would be it.

From: DColeman
To: CParnell
Date: 9/22/99 9:36am

Subject: stuff -reply -reply -reply -reply

Meet me at "our" place. If I'm not there in a few minutes come in after me—butt stuck in chair.

FIHH,
pps

From: DColeman
To: CParnell
Date: 9/24/99 9:21am
Subject: stuff

Mornin' glow-ree!!! Hit's Fry-dee!!!!!!!!!!!!!!!!!!!!!!!!!!!!!!!!! Cain't hardlee wait!! How are you today? I'm glorious! I got out and puttered around on the carport and driveway this beautiful morning. God is awesome! He certainly keeps things interesting.

I would certainly appreciate your help with my lunch and meds. What time do you eat lunch? I will work around you. For pp service from my pp sister, I'll call and tap on the phone. That bell is too loud to use. It screeches. Most unpleasant.

We were talking to Sam last night. As we went to bed we asked him when we would see him next—he is sooo busy, we have to ask. Well today he works at Kroger after school until 9, then he goes to catch the football game, then he goes to eat with his buddies and gets home around 11—we are already snugged in bed (us party animals). Saturday the church youth have Bulldawg tickets. He'll get up at 945, shower, dress, then race off. Again back around 11. Sunday morning we'll see him as we try not to be late for Sunday School. A year ago, this kid was a total homebody. If someone called him, "Yeah, uh-huh," were his part of the 30 second call.

Lastly, how do I get "notify" at the bottom bar on the computer?

Firmly in His Hands,
Debra C.

That'd be the University of Georgia Bulldawgs...as if there's any question.

From: DColeman
To: GWilliams, MBryant, JDieringer, AFitzgerald, and more...
Date: 9/24/99 9:31am
Subject: Friday challenge

No joke today gang. I left my copy at home next to the computer.

What I do have is a challenge. This weekend, hug one person you have never hugged before. At church, at the grocery store, at the hair dresser, at the ballpark (what a challenge in itself), next door, wherever you are. It may be a stranger or a "fringe" friend or someone you must forgive. Just see what it creates. Monday send me your stories. I love you all so berry, berry much!

Firmly in His Hands,
Debra C.

I don't know if she realized it, but between the jokes she would send out and messages like this, Dink was becoming the heart and soul of NGH. When it was time for her to stop working, the hospital administration would have been well advised to provide a means by which she could have gotten into their intra-net from home, because they lost a lot more than a good nurse when she left. I know her friends there miss hearing from her just like I do.

From: DColeman
To: CParnell
Date: 9/24/99 9:44am
Subject: stuff -reply -reply

Is 1 or 1:30 okay?

And no! We don't stay up til 11. Yawns start at 8:30.

FIHH,
DC

From: DColeman
To: CParnell
Date: 9/24/99 1:01pm

Did you get to eat or go to the bathroom just past 12:30 when everybody decided they needed you right then?

FIHH,
Slopoke

From: DColeman
To: CParnell
Date: 9/24/99 1:51pm

I'm just seeing if you are in your office paying attention or shamelessly socializing. If you're there, could you help me get up? I need to go over to Medical Records.
DC @ 1355

From: DColeman
To: CParnell
Date: 9/28/99 l0:0lam

Hey Smother Smister,
Thanks for your help yesterday. What an awful day! Satan is after me. I was so demoralized yesterday. First with the fall and then with the clothes switcheroo. When you called last night, Alan was on the floor beside my chair leaning on my shoulder and holding my arm and hand. He usually gets more smotherly after I fall, but this was so much more. To add to his concerns, I was really tentative and slow in my walking because I too am tentative after I fall. I suspect some of his was knowing that Catfish Hunter, a retired pitcher and ALSer, had fallen recently and struck his head on something and suffered a fatal brain injury. Frankly, I know Catfish was very distraught about his weakening arms so I know he couldn't take other problems an ALSer faces.

We are starting a male caregivers support group at our church in October. Alan so needs this and I talked to our pastor then talked to our previous, retired pastor about leading it—Jack Wilson, whose wife, Carolyn, has had a heart attack and breast cancer. I think he will be great. So I got Jack and Alan together and they took off running. There are loads of support groups around, but this area is very unique I think. I hope to start other support groups under the umbrella title of "The Barnabas Project." What do you think? Actually, Larry might benefit regarding his mother and her dependence on him. Do you think so? Anyway I worry so much about Alan. He was so pent up later last night and this morning. I may talk to Jack about pre-group counseling with Alan.

Oh it's raining again. Wasn't yesterday absolutely glorious? Praise God from whom our blessings flow. Amen and Amen!!

Firmly in His Hands,
DC

The morning before she wrote this I got a call at school from Catherine Parnell. She said, "Debra's okay. In fact, she told me not to call you, but she's in the ER because she fell again." The most significant part of the phone call was "she told me not to call you." I knew from that statement Dink was not in immediate danger. I trusted our relationship and her medical expertise enough to know she would not try to hide anything urgent. I asked Catherine a few questions, assured her I would not "squeal" on her for calling me, and told her to give me a call if anything changed. Catherine did call back later to let me know Dink was out of the ER and back at her work station, but it didn't make me feel much better because I felt like I should have been there. It was one of those occasions when she needed me to feel like she did not need me to come rushing in to take care of her. I stayed at school through the end of the day but was completely ineffective.

When I got to the hospital to pick her up, she had her head down on her desk. I said, "I heard you had some excitement this morning."

She replied, "When did Catherine call you?"

I didn't answer.

She was wearing hospital issue scrubs because she had gotten blood all over her clothes. The bleeding had startled the first people who arrived to help her—within seconds after she fell—because it was already pooling where her head was lying on the floor. When they got her to the ER, the doctors discovered the blood was coming from a cut on her scalp, rather than from her ear which would have indicated some serious head trauma. The cut had been caused by the hair clip she was wearing. Dink explained later that the scalp has lots of blood vessels, so even a small cut can cause quick bleeding. Anyway, Catherine helped her change into the scrubs in the ER, then sent her clothes to housekeeping to be washed. It was a pretty big price to pay for laundry service.

I want you to do something uplifting. Reread her message and notice the change from "demoralized" in the first paragraph to "glorious" in the last. She absolutely refused to let herself stay down.

From: DColeman
To: CParnell
Date: 9/28/99 12:10pm
Subject: unnerwear

Katreen!
Whut kine uh bloomers wuz doz yew let me borrey? My beluved wuz shoked! Dey wuzunt lik any' uh my bloomers. Iz dat dee kine dat yew ware when yew wanna make yer hubby frisky? Woo-wee!! Yew shor kno howta. No wundr Larree iz allwayz smilin'.

Yors trulee,
Floppy Mae

I wud ask fer yew to teech me but my hubby all ways haz a smile too.

Her change of clothes after the fall the day before included some hospital issue, funky-fabric under pants. As I was changing her for bed that night I seem to remember saying something along the lines of "What the he..."

OCTOBER 1999

Piles and Piles of What?

From: DColeman
To: VRider
Date: 10/1/99 10:26am

Concern yourself not with this morning. It's over. We figured out the problem and fixed it. You were just trying to juggle all my flailing parts at one time. When I get my hand in that hold strap, I will go to my knees before I will fall.

Now, FORGET IT. I will. I can't fret on past stuff; it takes all my energy to focus on tomorrow. God has equipped me well for this. He forgives me so I can forgive myself. I was ready to quit, but you forced me to analyze the problem and we were successful! On a Friday! WOW!

I love you my sister.

Firmly in His Hands,
Debra C.

If you could make yourself ignore the obvious tragedy of Dink's physical condition, you could probably come up with a pretty funny comedy sketch about two hard-headed women—one patient and one caregiver—doing battle as they try to get the patient into a typical mini-van. Dink would relate stories to me about her and Vicky grappling, fumbling, zigging and zagging, often times out of synch with each other, heaving and hoeing, literally knocking heads and other body parts as they struggled to get Dink into the passenger seat. They would alternately laugh and cry, cooperate and resist, fail and prevail. Occasionally, they would even get "snippy" with each other, but every day they would work together until they achieved the task at hand. In so doing, they developed one of those special relationships that is tested and strengthened by fire. We should all be so lucky.

From: DColeman
To: GWilliams, BBeam, BMurray, MBryant, KConner, JDier…
Date: 10/4/99 9:42am
Subject: That's Retirement

This is a bit long, but wonderful mirth for a blessed gray day.

When the teacher asked her young charges to put down some thoughts about their recent vacations, here's the essay one of them read out:

"We visited Grandma and Grandpa. They used to live in a really big brick house up here, but then Grandpa got retarded and they moved to Florida. Now they live in a place with a lot of other retarded people.

They ride tricycles down there, and everybody wears name tags—I guess that's because they don't know who they are. They go to a big building called a wrecked hall, but if it was wrecked, they got it fixed because it's all right now. They play games and do exercises there, but they don't do them very well. There is a swimming pool there. They go into it and just stand there wearing their hats. I guess they don't know how to swim, either.

As you go to the park you see a doll house with a little man sitting in it. He watches everybody who comes in. When they can sneak out, they go to the beach and look for seashells they call 'dollars.'

My Grandma used to bake cookies and stuff, but I guess she forgot how. Nobody cooks, they just eat out. They eat the same thing every night: it's called 'early birds.'

Some of the people are so retarded they don't know how to cook at all, I guess. That's probably why my Grandma and Grandpa bring food into the wrecked hall. They call it 'pot luck.' My Grandma says Grandpa worked all his life and earned his retardment. I sure wish they would move back up here, but I guess the little man in the doll house won't let them out."

Smile! Laugh! Make it a wonderful day!

Firmly in His Hands,
DC

From: DColeman
To: CParnell
Date: 10/4/99 2:43pm

Hey ppps,
Yep it's that time again. When you talk with Kathy Gillespie, would you ask her to bring my pay slip down here? I don't think she reads her email. Thanks!

FIHH,
Debra C.

Kathy Gillespie is the clinical manager of the second floor at NGH. Kathy was Dink's immediate supervisor when she was first diagnosed. Being one of those people at the hospital that I can remember for as long as Dink worked there, Kathy was a great mentor and friend to Dink during her time at NGH. I can't count the number of times Dink said, "I don't know. Let me ask Kathy about that."

From: DColeman
To: QMcCoy, KGillespie, CParnell, VRider
Date: 10/4/99 4:53pm
Subject: ALS clinic day

FYI—fer ya'lls infermashun
I will be gone Friday, October 22, to attend the all day ALS clinic evaluation marathon.

Oh, by the way, I have three children and they all will be graduating in spring of 2001. Sara from Medical College of Ga, physical therapy division, Joe from University of Georgia with a "your guess is as good as mine" degree, and Sam will graduate from Newton High School. We are setting up the Coleman kids graduation presents fund. See ya!

Firmly in His Hands,
Debra Coleman

Dink was incredibly proud of the kids. Each one has very special talents and abilities and she loved seeing them develop. As we now approach the spring of 2001, there are a couple of changes that should be mentioned. Sara will actually graduate in December. If you ask her, she can tell you the exact date and time…she's ready to start her career and conclude living like a student. Joe is finishing up at Truett-McConnell this year and is not quite sure what he will do next. He's a lot like me: unsure of what he wants to be when he grows up. He's a fantastic percussionist and we always thought he should pursue that, but then we don't personally know as many starving musicians as he does. Sam will graduate from high school at the end of May and start college this fall. He's going to major in Christian Studies and go into a ministerial field, he's just not sure which one yet.

Throughout the disease we strove to not let ourselves fall into the hopelessness of regretting the future we would not have together. For the most part we were successful, but there were two words that would always bring tears to Dink's eyes: graduation and wedding. We had made peace with the fact that the days of our relationship were limited, but it was incredibly difficult to face the reality that she would not be here for the milestones of the kids' lives. She always believed the kids were her most significant contribution to the world and, to this day, I deeply regret the fact that she won't get to witness her legacy as the kids go on to make their own contributions to the world.

From: DColeman
To: KAdams, GWilliams, MBryant, KConner, JDieringer, R…
Date: 10/11/99 3:39pm

A little mirth for Monday. Enjoy!

Great truths about life that adults have learned:
    1. Raising teenagers is like nailing Jell-O to a tree.
    2. There is a lot to be thankful for if you take time to look for it. For example, I'm sitting here thinking how nice it is that wrinkles don't hurt.
    3. One reason to smile is that every seven minutes of every day, someone in an aerobics class pulls a hamstring.

4. The best way to keep kids at home is to make the home a pleasant atmosphere and let the air out of their tires.

5. Car sickness is the feeling you get when the monthly car payment is due.

6. Families are like fudge…mostly sweet with a few nuts.

7. Laughing helps. It's like jogging on the inside.

8. My mind not only wanders, sometimes it leaves completely.

9. If you remain calm, you just don't have all the facts.

10. You know you're getting old when you stoop to tie your shoes and wonder what else you can do while you're down there.

Firmly in His Hands,
DC

From: DColeman
To: KAdams, GWilliams, CBabb, BBeam, BMurray, MBryant,…
Date: 10/13/99 10:17am
Subject: Mirth

Ok. Bear with me. Two jokes in one week but I need to send this one out before I fergit it.

The seven dwarfs gave Snow White a camera. She spent the day taking pictures of the dwarfs and her favorite places. Excitedly she took the film in for one-day processing. She arrived the next day to find they were not in from the processor. The next day, same story. The manager expressed his deepest regret as Snow White began to cry.

The manager said, "It's okay, Snow White. Some day your PRINTS will come."

Yea, I know. Yuk. Yuk. Cornpone. But you smiled when you said that! Mission accomplished. I love you all. Email hug!!!

Firmly in His Hands,
DC

From: DColeman
To: CParnell
Date: 10/15/99 11:00am

Hey,
I was reviewing this ER visit of an 82–year–old lady, in with chest pain. They do a battery of tests and the Dr. has this very involved assessment. Then you see, "The patient doesn't want to be admitted. Wants to eat."

Sssssssscccccccrrrrrreeeeeaaaaaammmmmmmmm!!!!!!!!!!!!!!!!!!!!!!!!   (that was me)

Dink was very committed to the notion that patient comfort is as important as patient cure, especially with older patients. I can almost see her mind at work here thinking, "OK. Even if you do figure out this lady's medical problems, what are you going to do about it? She's 82 years old, for pete's sake, let's just make her feel *better."*

From: DColeman
To: KAdams, GWilliams, CBabb, BBeam, BMurray, MBryant,…
Date: 10/18/99 9:35am
Subject: Monday Mirth

Thanks to all my looney email friends, I am newly refreshed and loaded with yuk-yuks for ya'll!!

Every night Joe would go to the store, get a six-pack, bring it home, and drink while he watched TV. One night, as he finished his last beer, the doorbell rang. He stumbled to the door and found a six-foot cockroach standing there. The bug grabbed him by the collar and threw him across the room, then left. The next night, after Joe finished his fourth beer, the doorbell rang. He walked slowly to the door and found the same six–foot cockroach standing there. The big bug punched him in the stomach, then left. The next night, after he finished his first beer, the doorbell rang again. The same six–foot cockroach was standing there. This time he was kneed in the groin, and hit behind the ear as he doubled over in pain. Then the bug left. The fourth night Joe didn't drink at all. The doorbell rang. The cockroach was standing there. The bug beat the tar out of Joe and left him in a heap on the living room floor. The following day Joe went to see his doctor. He explained the events of the preceding four nights.

"What can I do?" he pleaded.

"Not much, I'm afraid," the doctor replied, "There's just a nasty bug going around."

Ha Ha, groan, yuk yuk. I love you all. Make it a sooper dooper Monday.

Firmly in His Hands,
Debra C.

From: DColeman
To: CParnell
Date: 10/18/99 12:34pm

Well, all the millennium watchers who want to be at the first place the New Year occurs have bumped us off Fiji during the dates Alan can get off. We could go a bit early but that would mess up my research injection. But after I cried, I came up with a better plan. All five of us on a ski trip out west in our own private cabin right on the slopes. If it works out, the kids will absolutely freak. We would go while they are on Christmas break. Of course I wouldn't ski. Just give me a warm fire, beautiful scenery, and a good book, and I am jes fine!

Well, I'll let you know if plan two works out.

Firmly in His Hands,
DC

This is one of the most awesome stories of our experience. Back in the summer of 1999, a casual friend of ours at church pulled me aside and told me he wanted to ask me something. Lee Durden was one of those people we "knew" at church, but had never really spent any time with socially. All we actually knew about him was that he and his wife were very nice people.

When he pulled me aside he said, "Alan, Lynn and I have felt for a while that we were being led to do something for you, but we couldn't quite figure out what it was. Well, after praying about it, we don't know why, but we feel like this is what we are supposed to do." Then he asked me this question, "Is there anywhere you think Debra would like to go or visit?" Of course, I immediately burst into tears because I knew this was something I could not do for Dink myself and I was so incredibly grateful for the offer.

After I regained my composure and collected my thoughts, I said, "Well, a couple of years ago she said something about going to Baltimore and spending some time on the waterfront. She read about that in a travel magazine and thought it would be pretty cool."

Lowering his head, as if imposed upon, Lee said in a somber voice, "Alan!"

I thought, "Oh no. Maybe I should have said Chattanooga or some other location closer to home and less expensive."

Lee continued bluntly, "Use your imagination!"

Ohmygoodness! "Let me get back to you," I replied.

I talked to Dink about Lee's proposal and after a few minutes of discussion she said, "My ultimate, no-holds-barred, if-money-were-no-issue dream would be the Figi Islands."

I said, "OK. Let's see if that's imaginative enough." I called Lee and said, "When you told me to use my imagination, exactly how much imagination did you mean?"

He replied, "Try me." When I told him Figi, he said, "Let me make a few phone calls." I couldn't believe it. A few days later he called me back and said, "What about seven days and nights at a beach front condo in Figi, during your Christmas break from school?"

I said, "Well, if that's the best you can..." No, actually I said, "That would be fantastic, Lee!" Then I hung up the phone and danced around the den as I told Dink what Lee had said. Well, as it turned out, every possible form of lodging in that part of the world had long been reserved because it is so close to the international date line and would be the first landfall on Earth to enter the New Millennium. When I told Dink about that obstacle, she thought for a few moments then came up with the idea of a shorter, domestic trip for all five of us rather than the longer trip abroad for just the two of us. We had always wanted to take the kids snow-skiing out West, but had never been able to afford it. Lee and Lynn Durden made a lifetime dream of ours come true and there will never be enough time in all of eternity for me to express our gratitude.

From: DColeman
To: CParnell
Date: 10/18/99 12:40pm

If yew ar Cat, does that make Larree a dog, mouse or jes a hareball?

From: DColeman
To: KAdams, GWilliams, CBabb, BBeam, BMurray, Bcc, Mbr...
Date: 10/19/99 9:24am
Subject: Tuesday Mirth, or is that Tuesday Tirth?

Hey ya' ll.
Today's yuk yuk is dedicated to Glenda Lane and her teams in Surgery and Outpatient.

Two little kids are in a hospital, lying on stretchers next to each other in the holding area. The first kid leans over and asks, "What are you in for?"

The second kid says, "I'm in here to get my tonsils out and I'm a little nervous."

The first kid says, "You've got nothing to worry about. I had that done when I was four. They put you to sleep, and when you wake up they give you lots of Jell-O and ice cream. It's a breeze!"

The second then asks, "What are you here for?"

The first kid says, "A circumcision."

And the second kid says, "Whoa, I had that done when I was born. I couldn't walk for a year!"

Okay. I saw that sly smile. Gotcha! I love you all.

Firmly in His Hands,
Debra C.

From: DColeman
To: CParnell
Date: 10/19/99 5:02pm

Hey sweet thang,
Thanks for being such a wonderful buddy yesterday. And any time you need a bb, just pretend I called and come on down and pluck me up. I'm ready!

You are such a special and great friend. Thank you, and all glory and praise to God for putting us together. I love you this ……… ………………………………….much!!

Firmly in His Hands,
DC

P.S. As your nickname is Cat, if you go to my hometown in South Ga, I am only known by my nickname, i.e. "Who's Debra?" There, I grew up as, and continue to be, "Dink." I was a small baby and my cousin started calling me "Dinky." It (thankfully) got shortened as I grew.

*As I have heard the story from her family through the years, she's holding
back here. After coming into the bedroom where Dink's diaper was being
changed, the cousin called her "Stinky Dinky." I got an elbow in the ribs
several times during our years together for divulging the "rest of the story."*

From: DColeman
To: KAdams, GWilliams, CBabb, BBeam, JBenford, BMurray…
Date: 10/20/99 9:32am
Subject: Wednesday Wirth

Hey ya'll,
Today and tomorrow we'll look at signs. No mirth Friday—I won't be
here—but I'll be back Monday, freshly armed for the challenge of creating new grooves in your laugh lines.

   -Plumber: "We repair what your husband fixed."
   -On the trucks of a local plumbing company in Pennsylvania:
"Don't sleep with a drip. Call your plumber."
   -At a tire shop in Milwaukee: "Invite us to your next blowout."
   -Door of a plastic surgeon's office: "Hello. Can we pick your
nose?"
   -Sign at the psychic's hotline: "Don't call us, we'll call you."
   -At a towing company: "We don't charge an arm and leg. We
want tows."
   -In a nonsmoking area: "If we see smoking, we'll assume you are
on fire and take appropriate action."
   -On maternity room door: "Push, Push, Push."
   -At an optometrists office: "If you don't see what you're looking
for, you've come to the right place."
   -In a podiatrist's office: "Time wounds all heels."
   -On a fence: "Salesman welcome. Dog food is expensive."

That's it for today. Make it a very fun day. I love you all.

Firmly in His Hands,
Debra C.

From: Carole *(Dink's sister)*
To: Dink
Date: Sat 23 Oct 1999 1:47 PM
Subject: It's me again, Margaret!

Hey there! Just a note to tell you and Al just how much I enjoyed spending the day and night with you guys. I really feel like they are taking good care of you in Charlotte. I was very impressed. Also I admire you and Al for taking your illness and turning it into a witness. I know God is going to really reward you two if he hasn't already. Please remember I love you both, and I am willing to come anytime to help out (and do your hair and make-up). Thanks for asking me to go with you.

I love you piles and piles,
Carole

From: Dink
To: Carole
Date: Saturday, October 23, 1999 5:39 PM
Subject: It's me again, TATER!

My blessing was having you there. Alan was making coffee then giving my meds and he said he already missed you. Me too…Sam camped out last night with Ben Wardlow and froze his little patooty. It was about 1am when we got to bed. We got up at 11am. Good sleep! Snuggled under two blankets. Moving slow but purposeful this…afternoon. I guess we are headed to Ashburn Saturday morning. Mom is all but verbally insisting. I don't blame her. It'll be good to see all of them. I've forwarded some stuff to Leslie. Hope she enjoys it. I love you all.

Firmly in His Hands,
Dink

It was indeed a blessing to have Carole on that trip to Charlotte. In doing Dink's hair and make-up, she probably saved us 30 minutes at the hotel when we were getting ready to go to the ALS Center. I just never could get the hang of doing her make-up. I can't remember if I have it included, but one time when responding to Carole's "I love you piles and piles," Dink asked, "Piles and piles of what?"

From: DColeman
To: KAdams, GWilliams, CBabb, BBeam, BMurray, Bcc, Mbr....
Date: 10/25/99 12:40pm
Subject: Monday Mirth

Sorry I didn't get back to ya'll Thursday. I was very busy and when I had a break to get on the 'puter, either Judy was on it or there were crowds of folks in here. But, I'm back today! Enjoy.

More signs:
        -At a car dealership: "The best way to get back on your feet—miss a car payment."
        -Outside a muffler shop: "No appointment necessary, we hear you coming."
        -In a veterinarian's office: "Be back in 5 minutes. Sit! Stay!"
        -At the electric company: "We would be de-lighted if you send in your bill. However if you don't, you will be."
        -In a restaurant window: "Don't stand there and be hungry. Come on in and get fed up."

-Inside a bowling alley: "Please be quiet. We need to hear a pin drop."

-In the front yard of a funeral home: "Drive carefully. We'll wait."

-In a counselor's office: "Growing old is mandatory. Growing wise is optional."

Come to think about it, the wisdom we gather by Friday is usually lost by Monday. Right? Well, ya'll have a glorious day! As for me, my husband's finger stroking my cheek, my son commenting on my record slow time using my walker (so he can't get around me), or just to gaze on this perfectly beautiful day God has laid out, and I am sure my day is glorious. I love you all!

Firmly in His Hands,
Debra C.

From: DColeman
To: VRider
Date: 10/26/99 8:42am

Hicki Slider!
My cumfert? *My* cumfert? How kin yew say that? Don't yew drive like a teenager runs fer milk wit hims Oreeos? Don't yew thro cawshun to thuh wind an slang me up in yor van? Or head first inta a truck whose seat is 20,000 feet above the ground?

Yeah, I knows yew hav my bestest intrest at hart. Yew jes caint hep yerseff. I lub yew, sis!

Firmly In His Hands, (wit my butt in Hicki's)
Floppy Mae

For as long as I knew Dink, she was one of those very conservative drivers...you know, the kind you hate to get stuck behind because they absolutely refuse to exceed the speed limit. She was also the kind of passenger that would drive you crazy when she wasn't driving. She was what I call a "pedal pusher." Any time she thought the brakes should be applied—which was basically any time there was a car in sight ahead of us—she would begin pushing the imaginary brake pedal on the passenger side of the car. I guess what I'm trying to say is that she was a bit squirrely any time she was in a car. Vicky, on the other hand, drives like a bat out of that really hot place we all hope to avoid. I assume Dink was taking issue here with an "apology" Vicky offered about her driving style, while also trying to let her know it was okay...sort of.

From: DColeman
Date: 10/26/99 09:05am
Subject: Hey ya'll. Enjoy!

A young boy, about eight years old, was at the corner "Mom and Pop" grocery picking out a pretty good sized box of laundry detergent. The grocer walked over, and trying to be friendly, asked the boy if he had a lot of laundry to do.

"Oh, no laundry," the boy said, "I'm going to wash my dog."

"But you shouldn't use this to wash your dog. It's very powerful and if you wash your dog in this, he'll get sick. In fact, it might even kill him." But the boy was not to be stopped and carried the detergent to the counter and paid for it, even as the grocer continued trying to talk him out of washing his dog. About a week later the boy was back in the store to buy some candy. The grocer asked the boy how his dog was doing.

"Oh, he died," the boy said.

The grocer, trying not to be an "I-told-you-so," said he was sorry the dog died but added, "I tried to tell you not to use that detergent on your dog."

"Well," the boy replied, "I don't think it was the detergent that killed him."

"Oh? What was it then?"

"I think it was the spin cycle."

OOOOOOO! Yuk! Yuk! Yuk! Ha, Ha, Gross! I love you all. Have a terrific Tuesday!

Firmly in His Hands,
Debra C.

From: DColeman
To: CParnell
Date: 10/26/99 12:04pm

It's me agin,
We took the long way to Charlotte this time. We went up I-85 then to Toccoa to pick up my goofy, beloved, slightly airheaded sister, Carole. She has a daughter, Leslie, 11yo, just like her, and twin 6yo boys, whooboy! Instead of a four hour trip up and back, it was six hours each way. Alan and I got home just after midnight Friday and slept till eleven Saturday morning.

The clinic day was good, but incredibly long. Good natured me intends to fire off a letter of grievances. We had noticed, and the clinic confirmed, weakness in my shoulders (my slump), more weakness in my right arm and thumb and index finger. Hips are really weak, as evidenced by my stumbles, but my thighs are holding on. They taught Alan shoulder exercises to improve my movement, suggested ways to accommodate my inability to lift things over my head—like a brush. I just sit where I can prop my elbow, tilt my head, and brush. They also have extension rods for things like that. The occupational therapists have far and away been the most helpful to me. I just love them, and think NGH does a disservice to the community by not contracting one here like we do speech therapists.

The OTs gave me one thing I'll bring in for you to guess what it is.

The best part came from Dr. John Lindblom, pulmonologist. After looking at my sleep study and blood gasses, he said I was great. Two others diagnosed about the same time as I was, are on Bipap. Of course the breathing problems are the killers of ALS patients.

They also taught us air stacking where, using an Ambu bag and mask, we overfill my lungs to allow me to better clear my lungs later on.

Well, that's most of it. Very tiring and leaves me emotionally and physically drained. I love you!

Firmly in His Hands,
Dink

Dink's sister, Beverly, is four years older than she is, and her brother, Benjy, is four years younger than she is. Benjy was four when Carole was born and Dink had developed quite a "middle child syndrome" by that time. She immediately adopted Carole as "MY baby" and they developed a very close relationship through the years. Over the course of the disease, as

Dink's condition worsened, their roles reversed with Carole becoming the "big sister caregiver." She went to Charlotte with us several times and actually took Dink to Charlotte for me one time when I couldn't go. On our last trip, she was with us, tending to Dink the whole way up there and back. I couldn't have made that trip without Carole because Dink was in need of so much care on the road.

For a long portion of the return trip, Dink laid across the back seat with her head in Carole's lap because she could not get comfortable in any other position. I know seeing Dink like that was hard on Carole, but I think it gave her a lifetime memory of returning some of the love Dink had shown her through the years. Carole and I have developed a special bond too, because she is the one in the family that did the most of that kind of caregiving. It's not that the others were in any way unwilling, it's just that Carole lives so much closer to us and was able to be here more often.

The mystery item the Occupational Therapists gave Dink was actually a "booty wiper." At least, that's what we called it. It looked rather medieval and didn't work particularly well, but it gave us a lot of laughs and served as an extremely effective conversation piece. You should have seen the poor OT trying to explain how to use it without getting too graphic or explicit in her demonstration. It was a hoot.

There was good news and bad news at every clinic. The bad news was always, "You're getting worse." The good news was always, "But you're still here and will be for a while." All-in-all, that was a pretty good balance.

Bipap is a breathing assistance device that is not as invasive as a ventilator. Basically, it uses a removable mask and a pump to force air into the lungs. Many ALS patients use Bipap as long as they can before subjecting themselves to the surgery and permanence of a ventilator.

From: DColeman
To: KAdams, GWilliams, HBanks, Cbabb, Bbeam, Bmurray…
Date: 10/27/99 9:50am
Subject: Wednesday Whoopiee!

This is too funny and, in some cases, so true!! It came from one of my ALS buddies.

A Woman's Random Thoughts
    -Insanity is my only means of relaxation.
    -Women over 50 don't have babies because they would lay them down and forget where they left them.
    -One of life's mysteries is how a 2 pound box of candy can make a woman gain 5 pounds.
    -My mind not only wanders, it sometimes leaves me completely.
    -The best way to forget all your troubles is to wear tight shoes.
    -The nice part about living in a small town is that when you don't know what you're doing, someone else does.
    -The older you get, the tougher it is to lose weight because by then, your body and your fat are good friends.
    -Just when I think I understand everything, I regain consciousness.
    -Amazing! You hang something in your closet for a while and it shrinks two sizes.

This is pretty long so I'll break it up and send the rest tomorrow. Make it a wondiferous Wednesday! I love you all.

Firmly in His Hands,
Debra C.

From: DColeman
To: KAdams, GWilliams, CBabb, BBeam, BMurray, Bcc, Mbr...
Date: 10/28/99 9:35am
Subject: Terrific Thursday

Mornin' all you glow-rees!! Time for mirth.

Last half of "Random Thoughts of a Woman." Enjoy!

    -Skinny people can irritate me! Especially when they say things like, "You know? Sometimes I just forget to eat." Now I've forgotten my address, my mother's maiden name, and my keys, but I've never forgotten to eat!!

    -A friend of mine confused her Valium with her birth control pills. She had 14 kids, but she doesn't really care.

    -They keep telling us to get in touch with our bodies. Mine isn't that communicative but I heard from it the other day after I said, "Body, how'd you like to go to the six o'clock class in vigorous toning?" Clear as a bell my body said, "Listen witch...do it and die!"

    -I know what Victoria's Secret is. The secret is nobody older than thirty can fit into their stuff.

    -If men can run the world, why can't they stop wearing neckties? How intelligent is it to start the day by tying a noose around your neck?

Saying of the day:
Today's mighty oak is just yesterday's nut that held its ground. Bye all you nuts. I love you all!

Firmly in His Hands,
Debra C.

From: DColeman
To: KAdams, GWilliams, CBabb, BBeam, BMurray, Bcc, Mbr…
Date: 10/29/99 10:55am
Subject: Fridee Funnies

How-doo ya'll,
Are you like: Thank God it's Friday!!! or like: Thank God!! It's Friday.
Well, you both win. It's Fridee!! Enjoy the mirth today. It's dedicated to
those who encounter children during their life—that's all of us.

Whenever your kids are out of control, you can take comfort from the
thought that even God's omnipotence did not extend to God's kids.
After creating heaven and earth, God created Adam and Eve. And the
first thing He said was: "Don't."

"Don't what?" Adam replied.

"Don't eat the forbidden fruit," God said.

"Forbidden fruit? We got forbidden fruit? Hey, Eve, we got forbidden
fruit!"

"No way!"

"Yes way!"

"Don't eat that fruit!" said God.

"Why?"

"Because I am your father and I said so!" said God, wondering why he
hadn't stopped after making the elephants. A few minutes later God saw

his kids eating the forbidden fruit and was angry. "Didn't I tell you not to eat the fruit?" the First Parent asked.

"Uh-huh," Adam said.

"Then why did you?"

"I dunno," Eve answered.

"She started it!" Adam said.

"Did not!"

"Did too!"

"Did not!!"

Having had it with the two of them, God's punishment was that Adam and Eve should have children of their own. Thus the pattern was set and it has never changed. But there is reassurance in this story. If you have persistently and lovingly tried to give them wisdom and they haven't taken it, don't be hard on yourself. If God had trouble handling children, what makes you think it would be a piece of cake for you?

Thought for the day:
If you have a lot of tension and you get a headache, do what it says on the aspirin bottle: take two and keep away from children.

Okay. I must do a plug today. Chris Rice sings "Cartoon Hallelujahs" on his "A Night in Rocket Town" album. He is a great Christian singer and kids go crazy with this song. It's great!

Ya'll have a super Fridee and weekend!! I love you all!!

Firmly in His Hands,
Debra C.

A Nest of Dust Bunnies and Chewing Tobacco

From: DColeman
To: KAdams, GWilliams, CBabb, BBeam, BMurray, Bcc, Mbr…
Date: 11/2/99 12:21pm
Subject: Monday Mirth on Terrific Tuesday

Sorry I missed ya'll yesterday. The hectics caught up with me. This is lovingly dedicated to those wonderful ladies in Human Resources.

Sick Leave Policy

Sickness:
No excuses. We will no longer accept your Dr.'s statement as proof. We believe that if you are able to go to the doctor, you are able to come to work.

An operation:
We are no longer allowing this practice. We wish to discourage any thoughts that you may need an operation. We believe as long as you are an employee here, you will need all of whatever you have and should not consider having anything removed. We hired you as you are, and to

have anything removed would certainly make you less than we bargained for.

Death, other than your own:
This is no excuse for missing work. There is nothing you can do for them, and we are sure someone else can attend to the arrangements. However, if the funeral can be held in late afternoon, we will be glad to allow you to work through your lunch hour and then let you leave one hour early—provided your share of the work is ahead enough to keep the job going in your absence.

Your own death:
This will be accepted as an excuse. However, we require at least two weeks notice as we feel it is your duty to train your replacement.

Also:
Entirely too much time is being spent in the restroom. In the future, we will follow the practice of going in alphabetical order. For instance, those whose names begin with "A" will go from 8:00–8:15, and so on. If you are unable to go at your time, it will be necessary to wait until the next day when your time comes again.

All in fun. Hope you enjoyed that foray in the dysfunctional institution. I love you all. Have a blessed day and be a blessing to someone else.

Firmly in His Hands,
Debra C.

From: DColeman
To: CParnell
Date: 11/2/99 3:49pm

I LLLLLLLLLLLLLLLLLOOOOOOOOOOOOOOOVVVVVVVVVV
VVEEEEEEEEEEEE uuuuuuuuuuuuuuuuuuuuuuuuuuuuuuuuuuu
uuuuuuuuuuuuuuuu!!
!!
!!!

DCDCDCDCDCDCDCDCDCDCDCDCDCDCDCDCDCDCDCDC
DCDCDCDCDC
FIHHFIHHFIHHFIHHFIHHFIHHFIHHFIHHFIHHFIHHFIHH
FIHHFIHHFIHHFIHH

Hey Catherine, I do too!

From: DColeman
To: KAdams, CBabb, GWilliams, SBarbour, BBeam, BMurray…
Date: 11/4/99 9:52am
Subject : Turnday Mirth

Yep. Our minds are turning toward the weekend. Tomorrow is Fry-dee!!

This joke was sent to me by my cousin, Keith, who is currently stationed in Kuwait. Keith, also known as Skeeter, son of Marvin, also known as Bug. I have hundreds of cousins: Gel, Bennie Boy, Doodle Bug, June Bug, Dub, Cone…the list is endless, but to the funny stuff.

A young man named John received a parrot as a gift. The parrot had a bad attitude and an even worse vocabulary. Every word the parrot said was rude, obnoxious and laced with profanity. John tried and tried to change the bird's attitude by constantly saying polite words, playing soft music, and anything he could think of to set a good example. Nothing worked!

Finally John got fed up and yelled at the parrot. The bird yelled back. John shook the parrot and the bird got angrier and ruder. Finally, in a moment of desperation, John put the bird in the freezer.

For a few minutes, John heard the bird squawk and kick and scream. Then suddenly there was quiet. Not a peep for over a minute. Fearing he had hurt the bird, John quickly opened the freezer door.

The parrot calmly stepped out onto John's outstretched arm and said, "I believe I may have offended you with my rude language and actions. I am truly sorry, and I will do everything to correct my poor behavior."

John was astonished at the bird's change of attitude! As he was about to ask the parrot what had made such a dramatic change in his behavior, the parrot continued, "May I ask what the chicken did?"

Ha ha ha ha ha ha ha ha ha yuk yuk yuk yuk yuk yuk yuk ha!! I love you all. Make this day count.

Firmly in His Hands,
Debra C.

Dink's got me on the number of cousins with Southern nicknames, but I've got Ricky, Michael, Victoria, and Nicole'…who are siblings, also known as Ricky, Micky, Vicky, and Nicky, or collectively as "The Ickies."

From: DColeman
To: CParnell
Date: 11/5/99 11:03am

Confirmed last night. The 5 of us fly out Dec. 26 to White Fish, Montana. To a condo on the mountain where Alan and the kids ski right out the back door. I'm taking a good book, music, and my backed up prayers and plan to be the epitome of serenity wrapped warmly, sitting in front of a cozy fire. We told Sam last night. He was speechless. I guess we'll tell Joe and Sara this weekend. Sooooooo excited! Not as much as Alan though.

FIHH,
DC

Ultimately, the plans for the ski trip changed one more time. We ended up at Park City, Utah, in a ski-in/ski-out condo with a fireplace and a hot tub and a deck overlooking the mountains. It was wondermous. Thanks again, Lee and Lynn.

From: DColeman
To: KAdams, GWilliams, CBabb, SBarbour, BBeam, BMurray...
Date: 11/8/99 12:19pm
Subject: Monday's Mirth

Howdee ya'll. Wake up!

The Howl
The wolf man comes home one day from a long day at the office. "How was work?" his wife asks.

"Listen! I don't want to talk about work!" he shouts.

"Okay. Would you like to sit down and eat a nice home cooked meal?" she asks sweetly.

"Listen!" he shouts again, "I'm not hungry! I don't want to eat! All right! Is that all right with you? Can't I come home from work and just do my own thing without you forcing food down my throat? Huh?" At this moment, the wolf man started growling and throwing things around the apartment in a mad rage.

Looking out the window, his wife sees the full moon and says to herself, "Well, I guess it's that time of the month."

This is in honor of all those Monday growlers. I'll be back tomorrow. Til then—I love you!

Firmly in His Hands,
Debra C.

From: DColeman
To: KAdams, GWilliams, CBabb, HBanks, SBarbour, BBeam,…
Date: 11/9/99 9:56am
Subject: Terrific Tuesday

Howdy partners. Hope the week is shaping up just Dandy!

Sick at Church
A little girl was in church with her mother when she started feeling ill. "Mommy," she said, "Can we leave now?"

"No." her mother replied.

"Well, I think I have to throw up!"

"Then go out the front door and around to the back of the church and throw up behind a bush." After about 60 seconds, the little girl returned to her seat. "Did you throw up?" Mom asked.

"Yes."

"How could you have gone all the way to the back of the church and returned so quickly?"

"I didn't have to go out of the church, Mommy. They have a box next to the front door that says, 'For the Sick.'"

I know, I know. OOOOOO-yuk! This is dedicated to all those grandmothers prancing around here with a pocketbook full of pictures.

Firmly in His Hands,
Debra C.

From: DColeman
To: KGillespie, QMccoy, CParnell
Date: 11/9/99 4:07pm
Subject: DC's Disappearing Days

I will disappear Monday, November 22 & Tuesday the 23rd. It's time for my monthly BDNF injection. I will also disappear Monday, December 27 – Friday, December 31. Family trip. First in ten years. If you miss me I'll be in front of a fire looking out on snow covered mountains catching up on my serenity and my reading and my sleeping. By the way, if you know of any dynamite mysteries or good humorous books, let me know about them.

I know you'll miss me terribly, but you'll get over it.

Firmly in His Hands,
Debra Coleman

From: DColeman
To: CParnell
Date: 11/9/99 4:17pm

Catherine!!
I felt left out. You paged Judy, who left at 3:30, then Floris, then Kathy. I started to get them to page Catherine Parnell to 386.

Firmly in His Hands,
DC

From: DColeman
To: KGillespie, QMccoy, CParnell
Date: 11/9/99 4:26pm

Oops! Forgot. I'll be gone Friday, December 24, also.

FIHH,
DC

From: DColeman
To: KAdams, GWilliams, CBabb, HBanks, SBarbour, Bbeam,...
Date: 11/12/99 9:12am
Subject: Fridee Funnies

Mornin' all you glow-rees!
Fridee, Fridee in dee-dee do! Sorry I've missed a couple of days. My problem cup runneth over—know what I mean? But the mirth broke through this morning. Pardon me but you're going to get two family short, short stories, then a joke.

My 16 year old son, Sam, is nuts about cars. He's always saying he needs this or that for his car and his beat up old truck restoration. He works in the video dept. at Kroger. Alan was there last night when Sam called out to him and said, "I need ultimate speed stick."

Alan said he told him to get it. Now, Alan usually asks Sam if he has his own money for car parts. I was bum-fuzzled! After a few minutes I caught on. Duh! Gillette Ultimate Speed Stick Deodorant. Not a gear shift stick for his car! Double duh!

Then this morning Sam brought me to work for the first time. Bless his heart! Helping me get in the car, he did it backwards so my head ended up in his armpit. Thank Goodness for that Speed Stick!

Now this joke comes from my memory. My pile of jokes has been purged—either by me and I forgot, or the JCAHO twit fairy did it. Now I tell this joke with love. It's a blonde joke. My sister and nieces are blonde. Like all of us they show signs of brilliance and signs of duh-ville.

Here goes:
A beautiful blonde was tired of the dumb blonde stigma, so she decided to cut her hair and dye it brunette. That would do it! She went out and bought a sporty convertible and decided to take a drive into the country. She felt wonderful and "smart." She saw a shepherd herding his sheep along in a field. She stopped to watch. Suddenly she said, "If I can correctly guess how many sheep you have, could I have one of them?"

"Sure." said the shepherd.

"382." she ventured.

"Wow! That's exactly right! I'm impressed!" said the shepherd, "Pick out the one you want." And so she did.

Then the shepherd said, "If I can correctly guess your natural hair color, can I have my *DOG* back?"

I know! It's terrible. But so is my memory, and, I was blonde until I turned ten. It's in my blood. I love you all!! Have a terrific weekend. Drive safely. Hug someone. Be thankful for all these blessings we have received.

Firmly in His Hands,
Debra C.

The struggle to get Dink into Vicky's van every morning had finally over-whelmed the two of them. Vicky cried as she told me she didn't feel like she could get Dink to work anymore. Dink concurred, (and cried, too) so Sam became her designated driver. For the next month, Sam took his mother to work every morning on his way to school—in the same sleek Camaro Dink had reached for when she smashed her face on the carport floor.

From: DColeman
To: CParnell
Date: 11/12/99 10:29am
Subject: A number

Catherine my beloved beautiful sister,
This is an outdated telephone book. Jacob's Ladder Christian "stuff" store opened in April. The owner, Cary Wood, is a good friend but we talk per email. I don't know her number. It is imperative I get that number now! Hear me? Now! My sweet peach blossom friend.

Firmly in His Hands, (so he can't slap me)
DC

Apparently, Dink and Catherine just needed to chit chat occasionally. These next several messages fall into that category, so I'm not even going to try to comment on them.

From: Catherine Parnell
To: DColeman
Date: 11/12/99 10:47am

Do you think they found some dirt?

From: DColeman
To: CParnell
Date: 11/12/99 11:52am

Well, calling Jamie and Darryl, they either found dirt in the food or someone hated the food and threw a fit sending food everywhere, at which point said patient noticed a glob of eggs landed in a nest of dust bunnies and chewing tobacco.

Whatcha think?
DC

From: Catherine Parnell
To: DColeman
Date: 11/12/99 11:56am

I think I'm really not as hungry as I thought before checking email.

From: DColeman
To: CParnell
Date: 11/12/99 12:42pm

Oh, but think what creme brulee (sp?) looks like, yum!

From: DColeman
To: CParnell
Date: 11/12/99 2:33pm
Subject: One pup to another

Thanks for calling me a sick puppy instead of a demented old dog or just a weird old _art. I love you #@*='?!!

Firmly in His Hands,
Dink

DECEMBER 1999

Alan's Dropped Me Tons of Times

From: DColeman
To: Agnes Morehead; Amanda Fitzgerald; Arlin Hodges...
Date: 12/2/99 4:09pm
Subject: Thursday Tune-up

Hey all ya'll!!!
I'm back in the saddle so to speak. I've tried to stay out of Judy's way during JACHO pre-, intra-, and post tornado. I'm not fast enough to dive in and out of the computer area during her rounds. So let's get to it.

A dear friend sent this to me.
A man was walking home alone late one night when he hears a bump...bump...bump. Walking faster he looks back, and makes out the image of an upright coffin bouncing quickly behind him... faster...faster...bump...bump...bump. Terrified, the man begins to run towards his home, the coffin bouncing quickly behind him... faster...faster...bump...bump...bump. He runs up to his door, fumbles with his keys, opens the door, rushes in, slams and locks the door behind him. However, the coffin crashes through his door, with the lid of the coffin clapping...clappity-bump...clappity-bump...clappity-bump...on the heels of the terrified man. Rushing upstairs to the bathroom, the man locks himself in. His heart is pounding, his head is

reeling, his breath is coming in sobbing gasps. With a loud crash the coffin breaks down the door, bumping and clapping toward him. The man screams and reaches for something, anything…but all he can find is a bag of cough drops! Desperate, he throws the cough drops at the coffin and, of course, the coffin stops!

Dedicated to Cardiopulmonary and Nursing II who deal with the respiratory problematic patients this time of year. Ok. Now you can "Yuk-yuk-corny." I know, but cute.

On a personal note, my hair is now real short and real curly. A new phenomenon is happening. People hug me then play with and pat my hair. Brings to mind: am I a human chia pet?

Firmly in His Hands,
Debra C.

It was taking so long for me to get her ready in the mornings, we got her hair cut real short so I could wet it, comb it and go. Along with calling herself a human chia pet, she started telling everyone she had "Alan-proofed" her hair. I guess my styling skills just weren't "shey" enough for her.

From: DColeman
To: Catherine Parnell; Kathy Gillespie; Quinn McCoy
Date: 12/2/99 4:25pm
Subject: December ALS Clinic Days

I will be gone Dec. 20 and 21. Time for the monthly BDNF injection plus, this time I get to have a lumbar puncture. Simply can't wait!! But Dr. Rosenfeld's LP goes smooth as silk, but erectness is tough afterwards sometimes. See ya!

Firmly in His Hands,
Debra Coleman

"Lumbar puncture" is medical profession jargon for spinal tap. You remember those resultant headaches, right?

From: DColeman
To: CParnell
Date: 12/03/99 08:14am
Subject: OK, smarty britches,

Here's the rest of the story. It takes me a while to scoot from my side of the office to the computer. And the last few weeks Judy has been really busy. If I'm in her space, she is cramped and, in love, gets a bit testy. So, with JCAHO coming, being here, and her catching up what was put on hold, she is a bit more anxious, so I decided to avoid pushing any buttons and, groupwise, was down until yesterday and you got a joke yesterday. So there! Now, if you will kindly help me pull my pants down, then keep me from falling, I'll allow you to kiss my ***. Then I'll need help pulling my pants back up.

iiiiiiiiiiiiiiiiiiiiiiiiiiiiiiiiiiiiiiiiiiiiiiiiiiiiiiiiiiiiiiiiiiiiiiiiiiiiiiiiiiiiiiiiiiii
lllllllllllllllllllllllllllloooooooooooooooovvvvvvvvvvvvvvvveeeeeeeeeeeeeeeeeeeee
uuuuuuuuuuuuuuuuuuuuuuuuuuuuuuuuuuuuuuuuuuuuuuuuuuuuuuuuuuuuu
uuuuuuu

Firmly in His Hands,
Dink

I guess Dink was responding to a "smarty britches" remark Catherine made about the lack of email jokes over the past two weeks. Can you say, "Cat fight?" All in love, of course.

From: Catherine Parnell
To: DColeman
Date: 12/03/99 08:19am
Subject: She's back!! @#%!!!

Fussing at me may cause incredible wedgies!

From: DColeman
To: Catherine Parnell
Date: 12/3/99 8:33am
Subject: re: Fussing at DC re-butt-al

You can count on it, honey!

From: DColeman
To: Agnes Morehead; Arlin Hodges; Becky Beavers; Bi…
Date: 12/3/99 8:46am
Subject: Fridee Folly

It's here! Glory! About time!
Three friends were fishing. It happened that one man was a priest, one was a rabbi, and one was a Baptist preacher. The subject of when life begins came up. The priest said, "Why life begins on conception."

The rabbi challenged him saying, "Life begins at birth." They looked at the Baptist preacher and asked him the question.

The preacher responded, "Life begins when the kids leave and the dog dies."

Amen! Except we may fight with our youngest, Sam—16, over our over-sized smelly mutt, "Max."

Well have a good, no, a great, joyous, blessed weekend! I love you all!

Firmly in His Hands,
Debra C.

From: DColeman
To: Agnes Morehead; Arlin Hodges; Becky Beavers…
Date: 12/6/99 5:07pm
Subject: Monday Mirth

Hey ya'll,
I hope your weekend went just like you wanted or needed. Time to get back into the "swang" of things.

The Stethoscope
A nurse on a pediatric ward, before listening to the little ones' chests would plug the stethoscope into their ears and let them listen to their own hearts. Their eyes would always light up with awe. But she never got a response to equal 4–year–old David's. She placed the disk over his heart. "Listen," she said, "What do you suppose that is?"

He drew his eyebrows together in a puzzled line and looked up—as if lost in the mystery of the strange tap-tap-tapping deep in his chest. Then his face broke out in a wondrous grin. "Is that Jesus knocking?" he asked.

Ahhhhhhhhhhhhhhh awwwwwwwwwwwwww

Isn't that sweet? I had one more but my hunk of a honey bunny is here. Priorities, you know. See ya tomorrow. I love you all!!!!

Firmly in His Hands,
Debra C.

From: DColeman
To: Agnes Morehead; Arlin Hodges; Becky Beavers…
Date: 12/7/99 12:38pm
Subject: Tuesday Tickler

Howdee do ya'll,
Any froze' nose 'n toes out there? Well, let me get you laughing.

A child came home from Sunday School and told his mother he had learned a new song about a cross-eyed bear named gladly. It took his mother awhile before she realized the hymn was really "Gladly, The Cross I'd Bear."

One summer evening during a violent thunderstorm a mother was tucking her small son into bed. She was about to turn off the light when he asked with a tremor in his voice, "Mommy, will you sleep with me tonight?" The mother smiled and gave him a reassuring hug.

"I can't, dear," she said. "I have to sleep in Daddy's room."

A long silence was broken at last by his shaky little voice, "The big sissy."

Little kids are just precious—sometimes. Have a super day. I love you all!

Firmly in His Hands,
Debra C.

From: DColeman
To: CParnell
Date: 12/7/99 12:57pm
Subject: Nothing in Particular

Hey sweetie sister,
You look very red and black today. I would venture to say you have no
pink in your wardrobe. The first electric wheelchair the GA ALS Assn.
brought by for me to use developed a wiring problem and I couldn't use
it. That was a couple of months ago. Last night they swapped that one
with a bigger one that tilts back so I can relieve butt spots. Alan is in the
process of refinancing the house to help with redoing our bathroom
and other projects. And then we'll get a van and get it converted. Sam
says he can't wait! He says I get heavier and heavier each
morning…until I give him the evil eye—then he breaks into his heart
melting grin.

I got together with Rev. Jack Wilson and Alan and told them about my
idea for a male care givers support group. They picked up the ball. We
have a core group to start with then we'll expand into support groups
for other stuff. I have named it "The Barnabas Project."

Well, gotta go. Judy's back. I love you!!!

Firmly in His Hands,
Debra C.

We never could seem to get it together on a power wheelchair. The new one
she refers to here was actually useless because it had a very sensitive joy-
stick control. Since she had lost most of her fine motor skills, she couldn't
apply the correct finesse to operate it. She nearly slung herself out of it one
time and had a very difficult time navigating down the hall and around

the corner into our bedroom. Like I said earlier, I wish I had resolved this issue a lot earlier in the disease.

The Barnabas Project finally came together in December. Dink was very pleased with all aspects of it, except when Jack Wilson tried to identify it as the "Debra Coleman Caregivers Support Group." She wanted no part of having her name included in the title and made that fact VERY clear to Jack and myself. We obliged her with the name change…quickly.

From: Carole
To: Dink
Date: Tues 7 Dec 1999 3:50 PM
Subject: Hello

Hey Dink!
I thought I'd drop you a line to see how your weekend went with Joyce. I know the ladies in your church had a wonderful experience. What all did you do? How are you? Have you recovered from our big adventure? I hope I didn't hurt you. I guess I just need to come over and get some more experience. Let me know how you are. I've really been thinking about you lately.

Love you a lot!
Carole

From: Dink
To: Carole
Date: Tue December 07, 1999 6:23 PM
Subject: Re: Hello

Hey Tater,
We had such a blessing from God through Joyce. One thing she said was, "Don't tell God how big your problems are. Tell your problems

how big your God is." She was great! Are you going to her January retreat in Toccoa?

No, you didn't hurt me in Charlotte. We're laughing about it. Yep, we failed to train you. And the lady at the clinic was awful. To walk, I need to waddle to help pick up my feet. She was holding my waist so tightly, no waddle, no walk.

I'm over the overwhelming frustration, not because of anyone, just because of the problems of ALS. Don't fret. Alan's dropped me tons of times.

I hope ya'll are doing fine. Say, do the kids like Veggie Tales? Do they have any of the videos? Well, I need to run. (Get it? Run? Me? yuk yuk)

I love you.

Firmly in His Hands,
Dink

Joyce Payne is a Methodist minister who, for years, has lead a ladies summer retreat for a group of women from Ashburn (Dink's hometown). Dink attended the retreat in May of 1999 and later asked Joyce to lead one in Covington. After making sure it was okay with our Baptist minister, Dink booked Joyce for a one-day ladies retreat at our church on December 4, 1999. Using email and faxes, she organized the entire event and wound up with a dozen women in attendance, including a few from other churches. By all accounts, it was a rousing success.

From: DColeman
To: AMorehead; AHodges; BBeavers…
Date: 12/8/99 1:58pm

Subject: Wednesday Winkles

Hey gang!
Isn't this a beeyooteefull day!!?? I could get lost in the glorious blue of the sky this morning! Well let's get right to the mirth.

Nine year old Joey was asked by his mother what he had learned in Sunday School. "Well, Mom, our teacher told us how God sent Moses behind enemy lines on a rescue mission to lead the Israelites out of Egypt. When he got to the Red Sea, he had his engineers build a pontoon bridge, and all the people walked across safely. Then he used his walkie talkie to radio headquarters and call in an air strike. They sent in bombers to blow up the bridge and all the Israelites were saved."

"Now, Joey, is that really what your teacher taught you?" his mother asked.

"Well, no, Mom, but if I told it the way the teacher did, you'd never believe it!"

A four year old Catholic boy and a four year old Protestant girl were playing in a plastic wading pool in the back yard. They splashed a lot of water on each other. Their clothes got soaking wet so they decided to take them off. The little boy looked at the little girl and said, "Golly, I didn't know there was that much difference between Catholics and Protestants."

Hang in there. Two more days. Smile! I love you all!!

Firmly in His Hands,
Debra C.

Unfortunately, there were not "two more days." In fact, there were no more days. This is the last email she wrote at NGH and it turned out to be her last day at work as well. Neither "last" had been planned as such.

About four o'clock on the afternoon of Wednesday, December 8, I got a call from the Human Resources director at NGH. He said, "Alan, we need to meet with you and Debra. When can you come in?" I told him I had to work every day and it would be the next week before I could arrange some time off. He said, "We really need to meet tomorrow." He persisted and I relented so we made an appointment for 9:00 the next morning.

Dink heard the conversation and realized who I was talking to. When I hung up the phone and looked at her she was crying and pounding away on her LightWriter, "I WILL NOT LET THEM FORCE ME TO QUIT!" Her eyes were glaring in a way that confirmed she would not negotiate that point.

Wanting to refocus all of the emotion I could see on her face, I said, "Well, work on your argument and get it bullet-proof so we'll be prepared tomorrow." I don't remember how much planning she did for the next morning's meeting, but I do remember neither of us could sleep much that night.

When we got to the hospital on Thursday morning we met with the HR director and the Nursing Services director. Dink was incredibly tense as I wheeled her into the office and got her situated, but she was "loaded for bear" and ready to fight it out. Knowing Dink as they did, though, the managers were very shrewd. They told us the emotional and physical strain on the people who worked closest to Dink (and therefore were her primary caregivers at the hospital) was beginning to effect the caregivers' ability to perform their other duties. Dink immediately softened. In fact, she didn't even ask any questions for clarification because she was more adamant about not burdening her friends at work than she was about staying on the job. We listened distantly as the managers explained the details about the separation of service, then we all cried, and I took her back home. It was a long, silent drive.

CHRISTMAS 1999

I'll Be Right Back

True to her resilient nature, Dink immediately refocused her energy on planning for Christmas and the ski trip. We went to Ashburn for Christmas but only stayed one night because she couldn't get comfortable in the chairs and beds at her parents' home. When we left, I think we both new it was her last visit down there.

Leaving for the ski trip on December 26 was interesting too. We had to take two cars to get all of our belongings to the airport, so Sara's boyfriend, James, provided taxi service for us. Sara, Joe and James took the cars to the parking deck after dropping off Dink, Sam, and me at the check-in curb so we could head on down to the plane. When the three of us got to the boarding gate we realized Sara had all of our identification and tickets because she checked all the luggage. After declaring she wasn't supposed to, the boarding agent allowed us to board the plane early—without tickets—since it would take so long to get Dink to her seat. In the mean time, after cutting off a big SUV to get a parking spot, Joe couldn't get the power window on the driver's side of my car to go up. He was going to leave it down, but Sara objected, so in the middle of having a mini-fight, they managed to get the window up. Then they had to dash through the airport to arrive at the gate just as the boarding agents made the final call to board. There's nothing quite like a calm, smooth start to a vacation, is there? But it was worth it.

Obviously that was our first and only experience flying while Dink was sick, but I have to say, the travel industry could make a TON of improvements for people with mobility challenges. We were totally displeased with the service we received. The approach of the airline seemed to be "OK, let's see how we can get her seated with the least effort on our part." On the flight to Salt Lake City, the head flight attendant did reassign us to the first seat behind the first class section, which provided more room for me to work with Dink during the flight, but on the return flight, another attendant refused to do so. In fact, he wouldn't even move her to the aisle seat of our row, so we ended up manhandling her across two seats to get to our assigned seats. It was miserable. I know we're talking here about a business that lives and dies by seat occupancy, but it seams to me they could give up one seat per plane to allow for enough room to accommodate someone in a wheelchair. Bless her heart, Sara got pro-active with the issue, firing off a couple of scathing letters to Delta. Their response? They sent us discount vouchers so we could experience the indignation all over again...but for less money. I never could bring myself to use them.

That's enough negativity.

The time in Park City, Utah, was terrific. We actually had all five of us together for five days, in the same condo, with virtually no arguing. For our headstrong bunch, that was a world record in itself. It was the first time the kids had skied out west, and even with forty percent of the slopes closed, there was more snow on the ground than they had ever seen at one place before. We developed an informal daily schedule that worked out great. The kids would head out to the slopes immediately after breakfast while I got Dink dressed and ready for the day. Then, when I was ready to head out myself, one of them would come in for a break and hang out with her for a while. We just rotated through the day like that. There were a few times we were all on the slopes at the same time, but that was okay with Dink because it gave her a chance to enjoy the quiet and do some reading.

We had a bathroom-funny at the condo, too. The commode closet in the master suite was extremely small so I had to remove its door to be able to get Dink in there. After she would finish her business, I would stand her up, then, because there was so little room to maneuver, I had to step around behind her to help her walk back to her chair. One time, just as I got into position, she lost her balance and we both fell back-wards and landed on the commode with her in my lap. Of course we cracked up and couldn't quit laughing for several minutes, but then I realized I couldn't stand up with her in my lap, which just brought on more laughter. When we finally regained our composure, I called out for Sam, but he was in the den watching television and the doors to our suite and our bathroom were both closed, so he couldn't hear me. Then I yelled out, "SAM!!!" This time he came running in with a frantic look on his face which turned into a big smile when he realized we were okay. I said, "Help us up, dude."

He raised his hand as if to say, "Just a moment," then he said, "I'll be right back." Of course, he came back in with his camera and wouldn't help us up until we let him take a picture, but we didn't object too seriously.

When Dink quit working in December, there were only a couple of weeks of school left until Christmas holidays started, so she stayed home by herself. I would set her up in the recliner with her Bible, another good book, and the remote control for the TV. I'd also put a movie in the VCR that she could watch if she wanted. There was one movie she watched almost daily and she would cry every time she watched it. I said, "Baby, you cry every time you watch this and you watch it every day...how many more times are you gonna watch it?"

"Until I can watch it without crying."

"Okay, dear."

I would come home each day at lunch to give her a potty break and feed her, make sure she had everything set up for the afternoon, including another movie if needed, then head back to school. That system worked fine for those ten or twelve days, but I knew I would have to make other arrangements for January. What I didn't know was the fact that those arrangements were already being made.

According to the Bible, your good works here on Earth don't get you into Heaven, but they do influence the size of your heavenly home. Ardis Young and Lynn Wojcik must have mansions beyond imagination waiting for them there. Ardis, calling on members of our church, and Lynn, calling on the staff at NGH, put together a team of volunteers that came in to sit with Dink when school resumed in January. They handled the entire matter: recruiting, scheduling and even training the ladies, whom we called "Dink's Angels." In fact, there were many days I would leave for school, not knowing who would be coming in that day. Some of the ladies were nurses, but many were not. Some took time off from work to come in. Some could come only for mornings, others only for afternoons and a few could stay the whole day. Once or twice, I came in at lunch and said, "Hi. I'm Alan. Who are you?" because I had never met that particular sitter. I never had to think twice about the entire operation because Ardis and Lynn were so dedicated and took total responsibility for everything from the very beginning. There's no telling how much money they saved us, and I can't even begin to estimate how much stress they personally eliminated from our lives. I wish I could express my gratitude but, as yet, I have not been authorized to create new words for the English language and that is exactly what it would take for me to have the right words to use. Ardis, Lynn and the rest of the "Angels"…my heart is eternally yours.

DINK'S VICTORY

I Actually Enjoyed That Service

January, February and March saw a steady and rapid progression of the disease. I don't need to recount any of it here, because it would read like any of a large number of textbooks dealing with the end stages of ALS. Basically, everything just quit working until one day, March 28, 2000, that included her lungs. This is what I wrote to friends about that day.

To a good friend who lives in Florida:

Sunday Apr 2, 2000
Hey dear, I have a phone in my office at school. It's the one I called you from several months ago when you paged me. It's in there primarily for the annual staff, which meets in my room during my planning period. A lot of times I don't even answer it because it's almost always for them. Tuesday morning it rang a few minutes after eight o'clock and the only reason I picked it up is because we are in the middle of doing parent conferences for registration and I had left messages with a couple of parents to call me back. The person on the line was talking to someone else when I picked up, saying, "I can't get an answer." When I said "Hello," she responded, "Alan, this is Cherry Rutland. It's an emergency. Debra's unconscious." I verified that she had called 911 then told her I would be right home. I came out of the office and headed straight toward the door at the back of the lab that leads out to the parking lot. I'm in a team teaching situation first period

and when I told the other teacher to take over, he said "GO!" As I raced home, I was agonizing over a thousand different thoughts. Of course, I knew this could be "it"...I wondered if she might have fallen from her chair again...I thought of what might happen if they revived her but injured her in the process...I was distraught at the idea that she had been alone...I wondered how we would manage if she had to go in the hospital for an extended time. But about half way home, a sense of awareness came over me and I knew she was gone. Almost all of the other thoughts left my head and I drove on in somewhat of a state of shock. When I got to the house, the paramedics, first responders, firefighters and sheriff's department were all here. I jumped out of the car almost before it was stopped and ran toward the house. I saw Rosemary Davenport, who is my next door neighbor and a firefighter, in the driveway and the look on her face confirmed what I was already expecting. I ran through the kitchen and into the den and found her lying on the floor in front of the place where her chair usually sits. (The chair had been moved, but I didn't even realize that until some time later.) She was partially covered by the white sheet and I remember thinking, "I wish I didn't have this picture in my mind." I knelt down on the floor beside her, stroked her face, held her hand, and sobbed uncontrollably. I remember telling her I hadn't wanted her to be alone and I thought we had more time. After some time I started taking her neck brace off and Cherry knelt down to help me. When it was off, her head rested back against the floor, completely relaxed. Her lips had lost their muscularity early in the disease and have hung limp and open for several months now, but when her head settled back against the floor, they fell into what can only be described as a sweet, small smile. Immediately, I knew everything was okay. I knew she was alright and it was the right time and she probably had even chosen the time. It was at that moment, when I realized she was comfortable again for the first time in months, that I was alright too. Of course, I'm grieving and missing her terribly, but I've got that deep down contentment and sense of peace. I know everything's okay.
Alan

To Mark and Marion Weaver, our clinic and study buddies from Sumter, South Carolina:

Hey guys,
This is Alan. I don't know if you've talked to anyone from Charlotte in the last several days so I wanted to share some news with you. On Tuesday morning, March 28, Dink beat the disease. She laid her head back against the chair she was sitting in, then quietly and peacefully gave up the fight. On her own terms, in her own time. Over the previous month our communication was limited to her writing imaginary letters in my palm. She had developed a twitch in her right hand in the last ten days, or so, and the palm writing had become increasingly difficult to decipher. She knew, and I knew, as bad as things have been the last two years, they were going to get a whole lot worse if we lost the ability to communicate. I firmly believe in my heart she decided it wouldn't be worth the fight if we couldn't "talk." So when her sitter for the day arrived less than 30 minutes after our son had left for school, Dink was already gone. No signs of struggle or discomfort, just peacefully sitting there as if asleep. She went the way we ALL have told people WE would like to go when it's our time. Her terms, her time, in her own home, in total victory. Our mantra the last few months has been: "Wellness is temporary, wholeness is eternal." I am so very proud of her and many times more than that, I am so very happy she is whole again. I'm OK now, cause I know she's OK now. I would much rather have talked with you guys in person about this, but more than that, I wanted to make sure you knew about her before you returned to Charlotte again.
You guys will remain in my prayers as we all stay…
Firmly in His Hands,
Alan

In the subject line for the email to the Weavers, I wrote "Dink's Victory." Her memorial services were nothing less than a Victory Celebration.

I had a number of people come up to me after the service in Covington (we had a service in Ashburn, too) and say, "Alan, this doesn't sound exactly right, but I actually *enjoyed* that service." All I could say was "Me too."

There was nothing sad about it because all we did was celebrate her life. Jack Wilson, who organized the Barnabas Project, started the service by saying there should be a large Smiley Face on her casket where some people put a family crest. He also related one of his favorite stories about Dink's wit and attitude.

> We came out of church with the Wilsons one Sunday when Dink was still using her walker. I asked her if she wanted me to go get the car from the back parking lot so she wouldn't have to walk so far. She shook her head negatively and started pecking away at the Lightwriter announcing, "Eat my dust!" Jack witnessed the exchange and howled with laughter, just as he did again from the pulpit.

When I woke up on the morning of the Covington service, I felt compelled to do something in the service to show the gratitude we felt for all of the help we received over the past two–and–a–half years. I knew there would be more people there than I could talk to personally, so I wrote something and asked Len Strozier, our current pastor, to read it for me. I had no idea it would be such an awesome moment. He introduced this by saying, "I want you to hear Alan's words:"

When we met for a while with Len yesterday, he kept telling us how today would be Dink's day. We would, of course, be worshiping and praising God, but it would be through the uplifting, remembering, and celebrating of her life. When I thought about this later though, something occurred to me. There's no way we can fully capture her spirit without honoring some other people, so I would like you to do something for me. It's a little different, so please bear with me.

If you ever came out to the house to sit with Dink, please stand up and remain standing.
If you ever sent or brought a meal out to our house, please stand up.
If you ever assisted her at the hospital, please stand up.
If you ever shared a financial gift with us, please stand up.
If you ever lifted us in prayer, please stand up.
(At this point, Len ad-libbed:) *If you ever had one of Dink's hugs, please stand up.*

Now everyone look around.

A lot of wonderful words have been shared with me about the witness and inspiration Dink and I have been to you. A lot of people have wondered how we could handle things as we did and have questioned whether they could do the same. But, I know you could. You would do it just as we did. You see, we didn't do it alone. What you see standing all over this sanctuary is the vehicle through which God gave us the strength to endure.

Thanks. Please be seated.

I'd like to paraphrase a story we're all familiar with. It's the one about the guy that's walking down the beach and he's been through a real tough time in his life. He looks behind himself, sees only one set of footprints in the sand and wonders why God has abandoned him. Jesus appears to him and says "You don't understand, those are MY footprints. I was carrying you."

When Dink got to the end of what she called "Our Great Adventure," and she looked down the beach behind her, she saw hundreds of footprints.

I will always be so amazed and so overwhelmed at the faithfulness you
showed as YOU carried us.
Alan

By the time Len finished reading the "*If you ever...*" statements, the
entire congregation was standing. It was overwhelming, not only to me,
but I think to everyone there. At that moment, we collectively realized
that we all had been part of a God-sized Victory.

Conclusion

Now I Can Answer Virginia's Question

This book had its origins in an attempt to answer the question, "How do you deal with your wife being gone?" I should probably address that question before I consider myself done here. There are numerous books on the subjects of loss and grief, all written by people with greater expertise than I have, so I won't even pretend to be able to address those topics sufficiently. What I would like to do is mention two things that have been meaningful and helpful to me. In keeping with the spirit of the rest of the book, I guess the best thing to do is to turn again to something that was written previously.

To: Alan
From: Carole

Hey Big Al,
I have a question. Did you and Dink purchase the "If there's a Will, there's an A" tape set? I thought at one time you had, but I might be thinking of someone else. If by chance you did, may we borrow it for a little bit? I've been told it has some great tips for "High I's" that can't remember stuff….like their names.

How have you been? Are you adjusting to a new routine? I'm sure you will have good and not so good days (as we have had). I really missed Dink when Matt broke his arm. She would have been the very first person I would have called asking for advice. That hit really hard. I do know she is keeping an eye on us. It's funny because this year Easter meant so much more than it ever has. It's good to know her life goes on even if she isn't here with us. I'm very happy she is singing and laughing and doing all the things she missed out on while she was sick. BUT...I can't help but miss her as I know you do too. Just remember we love you, and we are only a phone call away.

Love,
Carole

To: Carole
From: Alan

Hey Gang,
Sorry so long on the response...been kinda busy. The weekend was huge! Tons of fun for everybody. Sam was so tired Sunday morning. I had to have him on the south side of the county at 7:00AM to get on a van to go to the airport to fly to DC, after his getting in from prom 3–1/2 hours earlier. When the lady that was going to drive the van said "Load up!" he gave me a big hug and said, "Have a good trip." I said, "I'm just goin back to the house!" He was so confused. He probably won't realize he's in DC till Tuesday.

Yes. I do have "Where There's a Will..." and you can have it if I can find it! I'll let ya know how the search goes.

Joe's band was really good. If they had been giving awards, I would have gotten the one for Oldest Dude In The House...that was so strange...but lots of fun. The other guys in the band asked me if I would get up on stage if they could round up some timbales for me to play. I said only if they would play Soul Sacrifice by Santana...so maybe next time.

We are settling into a routine and it's getting more tolerable, except I'm having to relearn how to do everything. Either because Dink's not involved now or because it's just been so long since I've done whatever it is. I'll be honest with ya...I don't like it. One of the things I thought about that has helped, sounds kinda harsh at first, but when you think about it, it's just the way it oughta be. I keep feeling sad when something happens that I know she would have enjoyed being a part of. I find myself wishing it had happened before so she could be a part of it, or thinking, "What a shame she missed this." But one day it occurred to me: there's not a single thing here on earth, whether it involves me, or the kids, or you, or your folks, or anybody else, that if given a choice, she would choose to return here for, even if she could be 100% healthy again. In other words, NOTHING we can offer her here, can compare to what she's doing now. She'd turn us down in a heartbeat. After my ego recovered from that hit, I found the thought very comforting. But I do get lonely. Not that I'm counting or anything, but tonight will be the 35th night in a row I've slept alone. Ya know, even the last few nights of her life, though, after the lights were out, and we were all spooned up, in the last few minutes before drifting off to sleep, there was no ALS. We were like any other couple. It was the last bit of normalcy we had, but we had it till the very end. I am so thankful for that.

Well, this all got a lot deeper than I had expected! We're doing good ya'll. We're not rushing anything and we spend a lot of time together and talk about everything. We just need people to keep lifting us up, cause after 2–1/2 years of being totally propped up, we're not quite ready to stand on our own yet...and hopefully will never have to. Tell Matty-Mo to take it easy on that arm. Give the others hugs and kisses.

I love you.
Big Al

Another thing that was very helpful to my healing was the part I had in our community-wide Christmas Eve service at church. Len decided to put a different twist on the familiar Christmas Story that is often recited at such a service. He interrupted his reading of the second chapter of Matthew four times and had a member of the church relate a personal experience that paralleled the point of the story where Len had stopped reading. My turn came after verse twelve and my instructions were to address the issue of facing a significant reversal in your life. I started by reading my assigned verse.

Verse 12. And being warned of God in a dream that they should not return to Herod, the Wise Men departed into their own country another way.

The question you ask can never be "Why?" If you dwell on why, then there is nothing left to do but die. The question is ALWAYS, "What now?" Because asking "What now?" opens the door to hope and a sense of purpose on which you can focus.

My name is Alan Coleman and my wife's given name was Debra, but at a very young age she picked up the nickname Dink. In fact, if you go to the small town where she was raised and inquire about Debra and Alan, people will give you a confused look because they won't know who you're talking about. Down there, we're known as "Dink-n-Al," as if it were one, three-syllable name. I needed to explain that because people up here, who knew her as Debra, look at me with that same confused look when I talk about "Dink," which is the way I always refer to her.

So, after the Wise Men found the baby Jesus, God stepped in and said, "Time to go home boys, but you're gonna have take a different route than what you had planned." On January 14, 1998, we got a similar message from God. It wasn't in a dream. It was in the kind, but matter-of-fact words of a doctor at Emory. After a grueling three month diagnostic marathon, he confirmed that Dink had amyotrophic lateral sclerosis. It took me a week of practice just to learn how to say it. You've probably heard of it as Lou Gehrig's Disease. Of the many possibilities mentioned by the doctors over the past 3 months, ALS was the most ominous, so we had done some research on it. We found out it was degenerative, progressive, and terminal. We knew the average life expectancy was 3 to 5 years and that in the end, she would be totally dependent on others for everything. We were definitely starting down a different path than what we had planned. Within 6 months, she could no longer speak, nor eat by mouth. At the end of 1998, she began losing strength in her arms and shoulders. Spring of 1999 she began using a walking stick—she thought it was cooler than a cane—and by the fall of last year she was in a wheelchair. By mid-January of this year, she was 100% dependent on a caregiver.

Dink took the lead herself in making sure we kept our eyes on the big picture. She was writing to a friend at the hospital, chastising her for being so cautious and protective. She often called Catherine "Mother Hover" because she hovered over her so much. I want you to hear Dink's words.

To: Catherine
Re: stumbles.
My pastor has gone on and on about my being careful not to fall. I finally told him to hush! If I fall, I just fall. Not the end of the world. If I fall and am injured fatally, then I win. Glory sooner. You see, I am in a win-win situation. Now YOU hush!
Firmly In His Hands,
DC

Another thing we realized very early in the disease, was that the war we were fighting was won or lost in the daily battles. We found out quickly that we had to affirm, EVERY DAY, that "Today... WE are going to win." If we got cocky or proud or just lazy or forgetful, and we failed to make the affirmation, we would have a terrible day and lose that day. But we also realized the next day could be ours, if we would just claim it. We rarely lost two days in a row.

In July of this year, a young friend of mine who had lost a close friend of hers in a car accident, said to me "I miss Rob so much, how do you cope with losing your wife?" In attempting to answer her in a way that a 19–year–old could understand, I sent her a series of emails dealing with various aspects of her question. I soon realized that answering her was helping me more than it was helping her because of the way I had to think through my answers. This message to her reflects one of the key elements that allowed us to successfully endure what Dink called "Our Great Adventure."

Hey Virginia,

I'm gonna try to mix in some light and easy stuff with the heavy and diffi-cult stuff as I try to continue answering your question about me getting along after losing Dink. I hope you won't mind my continuing this cause I'm finding it quite helpful to me to think about this in a way that will allow me to answer your question. Maybe I should start laying down on a couch and calling you "Doc" when I think about this stuff. For the first year she was sick, there didn't seem to be any real evidence that she was sick except she couldn't talk. During the second year, when the large-muscle-group weaknesses started setting in, an amazing thing happened: people started showing up out of the woodwork to help and support us. The med-ical staff at the hospital where she worked (she was an RN) purchased an electronic communication device for her so she could "talk"…the hospital administration moved her into a quality control and chart auditing posi-tion so she could keep working after she could no longer communicate effectively with patients, families and doctors…members of our church started bringing us meals weekly (usually enuf that the leftovers would last until the next delivery)…a group at the hospital started covering the cost

of her meds, which ran around $1200 per month…a couple of pharmacists supplied us with the nutritional supplement she had to have…members of the church started randomly giving us money, sometimes $50, sometimes $500…the non-medical staff at the hospital took up a love offering and gave us over $4000…a group from the hospital business dept coordinated with a group from our church and held a joint yard sale and raised over $12,000 (that's not a typo) for us…a group of ladies from the church and a group of nurses volunteered and organized a sitting service for us when it got to the point she couldn't stay at home alone…even after she was gone, the church held a spaghetti dinner and raised another $4500 for us and then, on Mother's Day weekend, a huge group came out and re-roofed our house just because someone had noticed it needed to be replaced! The whole thing was absolutely overwhelming. So I guess this part could be summed up by saying we did not fight the disease alone and even now, our friends are keeping me and the kids completely propped up.
I hope you're having a great week,
Big Al

I tried to come up with an original summation of my ideas for tonight, but I kept coming back to some words I recently read in a book by Joe Martin, an ALS patient from Charlotte, NC. In the book, Joe quotes one of the preeminent ALS specialists in the country. The doctor admits he has no scientific or empirical proof to support this statement, but during his 20+ years of experience with the disease, he has realized three universal truths. I'll have to paraphrase his words slightly to allow them to fit our experience, but essentially, this is what he said: People who actively fight the disease with a positive attitude do better than people who take a passive approach. People who have help fighting the disease do better than people who face it alone. People with spiritual faith do better against the disease than people without faith. I believe this summation applies to anyone who is embarking on any path that he had not planned on taking. I believe if we had taken any other approach, we would not have won our battle with ALS, and I firmly believe that we did indeed win that battle.

Today is March 28, 2001. It's been a year since Dink's Victory Day and seven months since Virginia asked that innocent question. How would I answer her question today? In three parts. First, I have to get up every day and affirm that I will win that day, by eagerly seeking out the good things in that day and watching for signs of the good things to come in future days. Second, I keep myself surrounded by people who love and care for me, being mindful that the true gift of love is found in giving it back to others…and I have a huge love gift to give back. Third, I seek a daily, personal relationship with God, whose strength and love sustains me. And how do I do that? By remaining…

Firmly in His Hands,
Alan

Epilogue

A Final Word From Dink

The Carolinas ALS Connection is the monthly newsletter of the Carolinas ALS Center, located in Charlotte, NC. Each issue contains an interview article, titled "Patient Profile," and Dink was featured in June 1999. This is a copy of that profile.

Getting To Know Debra Coleman!
Debra Coleman grew up in a small town in South Georgia and currently works as a registered nurse at Newton General Hospital in Covington, GA. Prior to her diagnosis, she was a charge nurse on a busy medical unit while doing part-time teaching through the Education Department.

She married the "catch of the century," Alan, who teaches at Eagles Landing High School in Henry County, GA. They have three children: Sara, a graduate of the University of Georgia, who currently works for an ophthalmologist in Decatur; Joe, a student at Truett-McConnell College; and Sam, a sophomore at Newton County High School.

You were diagnosed with ALS in January 1998. What were your symptoms leading up to this diagnosis?
My symptoms really started in September 1997. At first, I started choking on liquids. Then I noticed I couldn't stop my exaggerated laugh to respond to the person or situation making me laugh. By the end of

October, my speech was a bit slower and slightly slurred. At this point, I knew something was wrong. After countless tests and many pokes and prods, I received the diagnosis that I had bulbar-onset ALS. Sixteen months after being diagnosed, my speech wasn't discernable except for "no" and "uh-huh." My lips are weak and, since ALS causes an increase in saliva production, this 43–year–old mother of three drools like a six–month–old baby who's getting new teeth!

How has your life changed as a result of ALS?
ALS has robbed me of my voice with its nuances and inflections. Now my voice comes from a machine that is lacking a southern accent and the quickness of my verbal response. I use a speaker-phone with my machine to talk on the phone, and I burn up the phone lines with email. But, at the end of the day, when I'm snuggled in my husband's arms, I can't whisper "I love you" or tell him about something funny that happened that day.

How would you respond to those that say you're "disabled?"
I'm still working at the hospital. As a charge nurse, I was constantly talking on the telephone or fielding questions from nurses, doctors, visitors, ancillary staff and patients. With my diminishing verbal ability, I had to leave that position. However, I've found plenty of opportunities for a nurse without a voice, but a fully functioning brain. My day is spent teaching in different departments in the hospital. I've had to change my way of teaching from verbal to visual, preprogrammed audio and tactile. So far, I've been pretty successful with small classes.

What has been your greatest source of strength and inspiration as you fight this disease?
My strength comes from my faith in God who, by His grace, will outfit me with a new body and joyous new voice one day. My husband, Alan, has been my rock here on Earth. He has been with me through all the

tests and doctor visits that left me crying as my future changed right in front of my eyes. Alan supports me with his love and acceptance of the journey we've begun with ALS. He and our children keep me focused on the good stuff. In addition, the people at our church and at work have been very supportive.

What advice would you give other PALS? (People with ALS)
Look forward to every day, every medication and every research trial with the highest hope and faith that this disease will be beaten. Having said that, keep one foot planted in reality so the progression of the disease doesn't catch you off guard. Access your extended support system—friends at work, church and in the community—to help you and your caregiver. Get out in the community and let others know about ALS. We need all the help we can get as we pursue a cure.

What has the Carolinas ALS Center meant to you?
I am inspired by those who are facing a life-threatening illness or permanent disability and continue to find joy in every day. You can see this very thing every time you visit the ALS Center. The joy is present in the waiting area as we visit, hug, cry and laugh together.

Any final thoughts?
Always search for the "pearl," the laugh, the joy, the love. Keep focused on the positive things. And lastly, when you see me, I need your hug!

Salutation Key

In keeping with the technological nature of the time in which we live, I decided to make this book "interactive." Dink had a habit of playing with her salutations by swapping around the first letters of the words they contained. For example, instead of writing "Hugs and Kisses," she would write "Kugs and Hisses." Sometimes they were easy to figure out like that, but other times they were not so simple. Here's where the interactivity comes in. Right after each salutation containing a letter switch, I've included blank lines where you can write the corrected salutation...if you can figure it out. Just for fun, I didn't correct any typos she might have made, so the first letters that appear might not always be the ones you need for the corrected salutation. I thought that would make things a little more challenging and interesting for you.

Lood huck and fave gun!   _____ _____ *and* _____ _____

Anywhere that two salutations appear on the same page, I have them listed here in the same order as they are on that page.

Above: Good luck and have fun!
Page 1: Hugs and Kisses.....with a typo!
Page 3: With wet kisses
Page 5: With hugs and smooches
Page 7: Back rubs & feet massage
Page 15: Snuggle Bunnies
Page 21: Hug and swack...........I don't know what a swack is either.

Page 24: Nuzzles and baby kisses

Page 25: Smooches and hugs

Page 26: Bear skin rug wishing.......If you got this one, I'm very impressed.

Page 32: Stretching and yawning

Page 35: Nips and snuggles..........A nip would be a small, romantic kiss.

Page 52: Slow as a snail

Page 54: Rub 'n' bubbles............She liked tandem bubble baths.

Page 56: Nagging Momma

Page 58: Running my fingers thru your hair

Page 61: Lubs and more lubs.........love and more love.

Page 62: Sleepless nights and sweet afternoon naps..........Another impressive one if you got it.

Page 63: Loves, snuggles and snibbles............snibbles?

Page 65: Rubs and slicky............she REALLY liked bubble baths.

Page 68: Lubs and painful butts

Page 69: Love and Hugs to All

Page 71: Sleepy and goofy

Page 72: Hugs and sneezes

Page 73: Lubs forever................got sneaky, didn't she?

Page 74: Cold toes and morning snuggles

Page 76: Sincerely from pain in the butt

Page 77: Rubs and snooches..................again I ask: snooches?

Page 81: Hugs and kisses.......without a typo.

Page 83: Lovingly, staggeringly, and woozy

Page 84: Hugless and goozy

Page 89: Broken snoz

Page 92: Cold toes forever

Page 93: All warm and cuddly

Page 97: Most breathlessly awaiting

Page 100: Love ya kid

Page 101: Listening to music and watching the birds

Page 103: Love for my hunk..................that'd be me.

0-595-22512-8